EXERCISE IN ACTION
YOGA

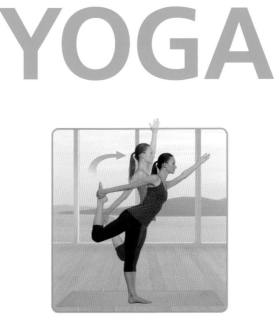

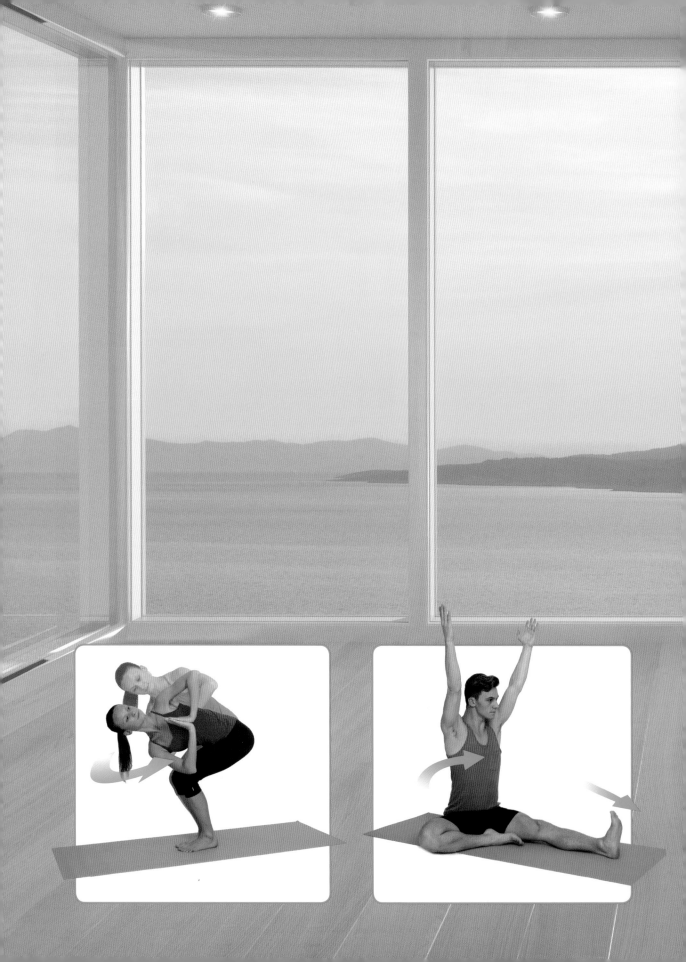

EXERCISE IN ACTION

YOGA

Betsy Kase

THUNDER BAY
P · R · E · S · S
San Diego, California

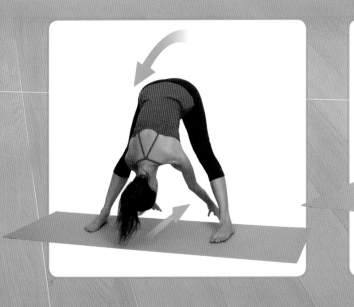

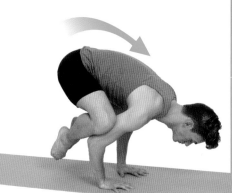

THUNDER BAY
P·R·E·S·S

Thunder Bay Press
An imprint of the Baker & Taylor Publishing Group
10350 Barnes Canyon Road, San Diego, CA 92121
www.thunderbaybooks.com

All notations of errors or omissions should be addressed to
Thunder Bay Press, Editorial Department, at the above address.
All other correspondence (author inquiries, permissions)
concerning the content of this book should be addressed to
Moseley Road, Inc., 123 Main Street, Irvington, NY 10533.
www.moseleyroad.com.

Library of Congress Cataloging-in-Publication Data

Kase, Betsy.
  Exercise in action: yoga / Betsy Kase.
    pages cm.
  ISBN-13: 978-1-62686-054-4 (pbk.)
  ISBN-10: 1-62686-054-8 ()
1. Yoga. I. Title.
  RA781.67.K36 2014
  613.7'046--dc23
                                        2013043437

Printed in China
1 2 3 4 5 18 17 16 15 14

CONTENTS

Introduction

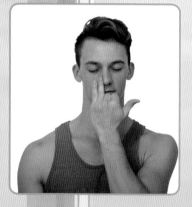

The simple act of listening, processing, and moving a part of the body breaks our preset tendencies, demanding us to be completely present. Can we draw our attention back over and over to the simple movements, the breath, and how this all makes us feel?

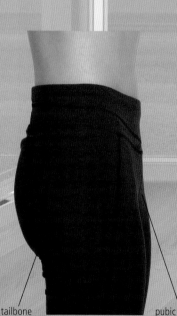

tailbone   pubic bone

Where are your pubic bone and tailbone? Awareness of these two points of your pelvis creates the ability to feel the placement of that part of your body whether standing or lying down in a pose.

What is Western yoga?

The yoga we practice in the West is very different from what was originally practiced not so long ago in the East. As Westerners, we tend to enter into the world of yoga through our bodies. We find ourselves drawn to a yoga class for physical reasons. Our sedentary lives make our bodies feel uncomfortable, as our muscles are tight and/or weak. The classes we walk into most often are fast-paced and flowy, sometimes with warm to hot temperatures, and are taught at our local gym or yoga studio. Students of all levels, and with different physical issues, come together to follow the instructions of a teacher. We begin to learn pose names like the Mountain pose and Warrior pose. We even begin to recognize the mystical language of Sanskrit, as the terms and pose names become more common. But many of these people find more than a good stretch in these classes. The attention to moving big and small muscles begins to set up the environment for a quieting of the mind to take place. The simple act of listening, processing, and moving a part of the body breaks our preset tendencies, demanding us to be completely present. Can we draw our attention back over and over to the simple movements, the breath, and how this all makes us feel? The body is the entry point into something bigger and greater than ourselves.

Anatomy 101

During class or when reading this book, you will hear directions that may need some explaining. Drawing your attention to specific places on your body creates better body awareness, keeps you safer, and focuses the mind. Most of us don't know where the basic landmarks are that we discuss in yoga.

Where are your pubic bone and tailbone? Awareness of these two points of your pelvis creates the ability to feel the placement of that part of your body whether standing or lying down in a pose. This is essential to keep the low back open and safe. Where are your sitting bones? These are the two bony places at the bottom of your buttocks when you sit on the floor. They are the base of your pelvis and are referred to many times in the directions to move in and out of poses. They are sometimes referred to as "sitz bones."

Where on my pelvis are my front hip points? These points are the two bony protrusions on the front of the pelvis on each side. Think about them as headlights on a car. When checking, ask yourself if they are balanced, even, and facing the same direction.

What does "draw your belly button to your spine" mean? This is another phrase you hear a lot. This direction is given to stabilize the low back and pelvis. There is no need to do a major abdominal squeeze here. Direct your focus to your belly button and a couple of inches below it, and see if you can engage muscles in that area. While doing this, you must be able to breathe. If your breathing is difficult, you are contracting too much.

sitting bone

The sitting bones are the base of your pelvis and are referred to many times in the directions to move in and out of poses.

"Draw your belly button to your spine" is a direction you hear a lot—it's given to stabilize the low back and pelvis.

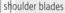
shoulder blades

The instruction to "draw your shoulder blades together" is actually directing you to engage the muscles between these two bones.

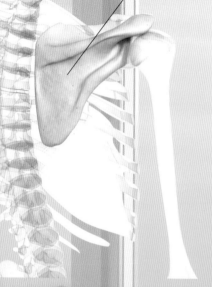

Most studios will have basic props, such as blocks, blankets, and straps, but you should bring your own mat when you go to a yoga class.

Where are my shoulder blades? These are the two triangular-shaped bones at the top of your back, behind your armpits. When you hear, "Draw the shoulder blades together," what we are really saying is to engage the muscles between these two bones. For healthy postural alignment, we need to build strength in this region to stand up tall and keep the chest open.

Props

When practicing yoga, you need a nonslip floor space. There are many yoga mats out there, but to start, there's no need to get too fancy. Your ability to grip the floor with your hands and feet is fundamental, so take off your socks!

When going to class, bring your own mat if you have one. Many studios will have basic props: blocks, blankets, and maybe straps. If you know you may need a blanket to sit up easier, or blocks for your lunges, invest in them. They are inexpensive and make a real difference in your practice. Remember, using props isn't cheating. Props can help you get into poses safely and with proper alignment.

Yoga class etiquette and clothing

Clothing can be anything that's comfortable and easy to move in. When taking public classes, remember that you are moving into all sorts of precarious positions—make sure you have the coverage you want! Also, have a layer to cover up with at the end for deep relaxation. Your body temperature will drop, and staying warm is important for relaxation.

When entering a class, there are things that you should be aware of. Make sure the class is the right level for you. If you are new to yoga, stick to the beginner classes. Try to get to class on time. Walking into class late is disruptive to other students and the teacher, plus you miss the centering and warm-ups. This part of class is really important to the practice, as is the end part when you get to relax in savasana (deep relaxation). Walking out before this part of class is a real disservice to you and your body. Savasana is the time to integrate the benefits of all that came before it. If you happen to walk in late or leave early (sometimes life gets in the way), be conscious of the noise you make, unroll/roll your mat quietly, and try not to disrupt anyone. Remember this may be someone's only quiet time all week. Be sensitive and respectful to everyone in the room.

Aches and pains

Should there be major sensations when practicing yoga? Moving the body in ways it hasn't moved before or in a long time sometimes creates strong sensations. What is important is to begin to develop a vocabulary to identify the type of sensation you may be having. The human body has different types of sensations: small and large stretches, pain and pleasure. Understanding the difference between a good stretch and what may be identified as pain can be challenging at first. Usually a stretch is not isolated to one very small area. Stretches are more generalized in an area or region of the body (such as the back of the legs). Pain is usually more localized, concentrated in one specific spot (such as deep inside the knee joint). It is important to understand that a muscle attaches at either end to bones. This spot on the muscle is actually called the tendon. The place we want to feel the stretch sensation is in the belly of the muscle, away from the two end points. Sensation at the tendon or inside a joint can mean you are stretching things that shouldn't stretch so much. Over time, this place can get "cranky" and can then cause injuries. If you have any doubt, ask an experienced yoga teacher to help you identify what it is you might be feeling.

We hope that, over time, the yoga poses become more comfortable and easier! Pleasurable sensations become apparent as your body becomes more supple and stronger.

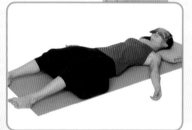

Savasana is a really important end to the class when you get into deep relaxation.

belly of the muscle

tendon

When you stretch, you should feel the stretch sensation in the center of the muscles. If you feel it at a tendon or a joint, you may be overstretching.

Movement/transitions in yoga and injuries

We have been hearing a lot about the injuries associated with yoga these days. We need to consider the many factors that may be contributing to these injuries. With any type of repetitive movement, there is always potential for injury. No one's body is absolutely symmetrical or in perfect alignment. The challenge is watching our habits and behaviors, developing a deeper awareness of how we move, and how it feels. Does it feel healthy in our body?

Many times, the actual injury that takes place in yoga happens during the transitions from one pose to the next. This is especially common in classes that move fast, where little direction is given to exit and enter into the next pose. Moving the spine quickly from a forward bend, to a back bend, to a twist, to a standing pose, to an arm balance, etc., puts stress on the muscles along the spine, and especially the ligaments and tendons that help hold the spine in place. Think about an expired credit card—you want to cut it up, so you bend it forward and back over and over again. What eventually happens is it breaks at that seam. Yoga brings strength and flexibility to your spine, so move slowly, be aware, and watch your transitions.

Yoga improves strength and flexibility throughout your body; to avoid overstressing your spine, move slowly through each pose.

Mindfulness and movement/transitions in yoga

There are three parts of any pose. The pose consists of the entrance into the pose, the pose itself, and the exit from the pose. All three parts should have equal importance and equal focus. To safely place your body in these shapes, the entrance into the pose should have a specific series of directions and full awareness. Once you are in the full expression of what that pose looks like for you, equal attention on holding it, breathing, and any sensations that may rise up need to be observed. As you begin to exit the pose, develop full awareness of what muscles you are going to need to use to support your exit, and where the energy is going to come from.

The concentration on these three parts of a pose continues to finely develop your awareness, stopping the distracting cyclical thoughts that we have running through our minds day and night. The mind slows down and clears out. Our nervous system begins to rebalance, and therefore all the other physiological systems (circulatory, respiratory, immune, and endocrine) also begin to rebalance. This snowball effect delivers better health, mood stabilization, increased energy, and overall positive effects on all the layers you are made of—physical, emotional, and psychological.

This is the "magic" of yoga. We start by moving, and then find ourselves at peace and stillness.

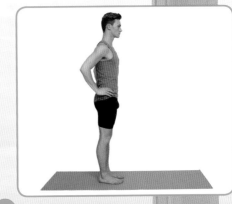

1 Establish your foundation, and bring awareness to your body and breathing.

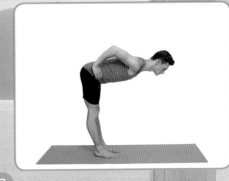

2 Continue to refine the pose, keep your breathing steady, and notice the sensations in your body.

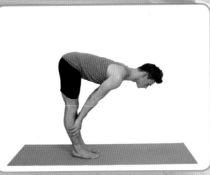

3 Reengage your foundation, press into your feet, draw your belly button into your spine, and lift up.

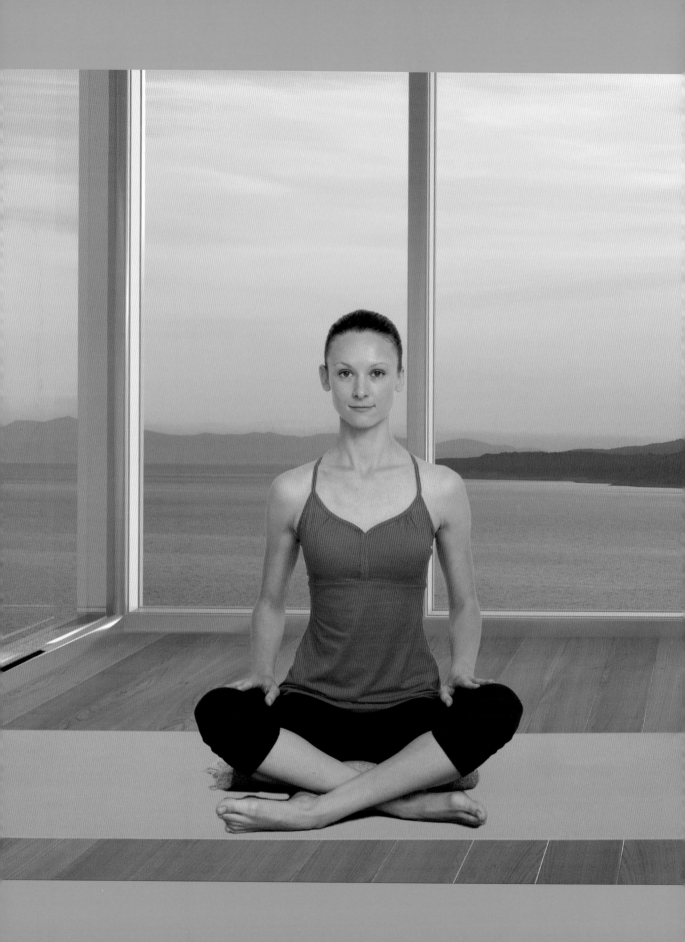

Centering and Warm-ups

Just as you would warm up a cold car before taking it out on a sub-zero day, you need to do the same for your body and mind. Centering allows for a moment in your day where you are still. This is the place where we can begin to notice how we actually feel that day. Warm-ups are smaller movements that move the spine in all directions: forward, back, side, and twists. Use this time to move your awareness inward. Turn the lights down, close your eyes, and get in touch with the physical sensations of your body, the rhythm of your breath, and your energy level. With practice, centering and warm-ups can have profound benefits physiologically, psychologically, and emotionally.

Easy Seat
Sukhasana

Sitting on the floor can be challenging. Over time, stretching and strengthening the body by incorporating yoga poses will enable you to sit more comfortably. If at first it is difficult, be patient—prop yourself up or lean against the wall to make it easier.

Step 1 Sit on a mat on the floor.

Step 2 Bend your knees, crossing your legs at the shins.

Step 3 Your knees should rest comfortably below your hips. Sit up on folded blankets if this alignment does not come naturally.

Step 4 Feel your buttock bones ground into the mat or blankets as you lift through the spine and crown of your head.

Step 5 Move your upper arms back to open your chest.

TARGET MUSCLES

trapezius

rhomboideus

erector spinae

multifidus spinae

SPINE

CAUTIONS
• If there is discomfort in your knees, place blocks or blankets to support the knees.

THINGS TO THINK ABOUT
• Adjust your position until you feel centered and balanced.

MODIFICATION

If you have tight hips, lower back, or hamstrings, sit on more blankets. If it is challenging to sit up, place the blanket up against a wall and sit back with the wall to support you.

Child's Pose
Balasana

The Child's pose is an excellent resting pose. You may place this pose at the beginning or the end of your session, or in between poses when you are flowing through a sun salutation. Think of it as your yoga time-out. The deep fold in the hips, the abdomen's contact with your thighs, and your forehead resting on the floor all enhance the level of relaxation.

Step 1 Start from the Table position. Press your hips back toward your heels. Rest your head on the floor, a block, or your hands.

Step 2 Arms can be extended forward, or crossed.

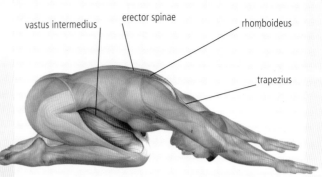

TARGET MUSCLES

vastus intermedius   erector spinae   rhomboideus

trapezius

ARMS AND BACK

CAUTIONS
- If your knees don't fold, don't force them.

THINGS TO THINK ABOUT
- When your belly rests on your thighs, the nervous system relaxes.

MODIFICATION

If your head doesn't reach the floor, place a folded blanket or block under your forehead.

1

2

Extended Puppy Pose
Uttana Shishosana

The Extended Puppy pose is a combination of the Child's pose and the Downward Dog (page 20). It is a great way to wake up the body and stretch out the back, lats, and armpits. Release toward the floor without overstretching the armpits, or sinking your lower back.

Step 1 Starting in the Table pose, walk your hands forward, with your fingers wide and your arms stretched.

Step 2 Press your hips back, lowering your chest toward the floor; keep drawing your arms back into your shoulder sockets. Your hips should stay over your knees. Relax your forehead on the floor, or on a block if it does not reach the floor.

MODIFICATION

If your forehead doesn't reach the floor, support it with a block or blanket.

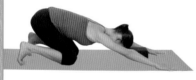

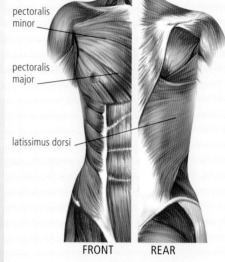

TARGET MUSCLES

pectoralis minor

pectoralis major

latissimus dorsi

FRONT   REAR

CHEST AND BACK

CAUTIONS
• Refrain from this exercise if you have shoulder pain.

THINGS TO THINK ABOUT
• Keep your lower ribs drawn in away from the floor.

Cat Pose/Dog Pose
Bidalasana/Bitasana

If you have only a few minutes, this simple vinyasa (to flow from pose to pose) is a great choice. Moving between flexion and extension keeps the spine supple and happy. It is also a great flow to coordinate breath and movement.

Step 1 Start from the Table pose, with your spine neutral, hands under your shoulders and knees under your hips, fingertips facing forward. Your shins should be parallel and your toes pointing back.

Step 2 Exhaling, curl your tailbone under, draw your belly button to the spine, tuck your chin, and look toward your knees.

Step 3 As you inhale, lift your tailbone, sink your spine, lift your head, and look up.

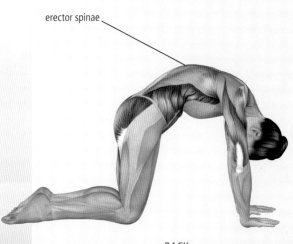

TARGET MUSCLES

erector spinae

BACK

THINGS TO THINK ABOUT
- Enjoy the coordination of the breath and the undulation of the spine. Close your eyes if possible.

1

3

Knees-to-Chest
Apanasana

You don't even need to get out of bed to do this pose. Any time you find yourself relaxing on your back, incorporate this pose. With the pull of gravity, the back, hip, and groin muscles get a great stretch with not much effort!

Step 1 Lie on your back.

Step 2 Exhale and draw both knees toward your chest. If you like, you can wrap your arms around your knees. With each exhale, gently draw your knees into your chest, releasing slightly with the inhale.

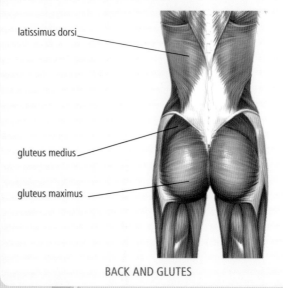

TARGET MUSCLES

latissimus dorsi

gluteus medius

gluteus maximus

BACK AND GLUTES

THINGS TO THINK ABOUT
• Experiment with your knees together and apart. The stretch will change.

Happy Baby Pose
Ananda Balasana

The Happy Baby pose is a little more challenging than Knees-to-Chest. By reaching your feet, your back and groin get a deeper stretch. If you can't reach both feet at the same time, do just one at a time. This pose is deeply relaxing and quieting to the brain.

Step 1 Lie on your back.

Step 2 Exhale and draw both knees toward your chest; unfold your knees and grab the inside arches of your feet with both hands.

Step 3 The soles of your feet should face the ceiling; your knees move down under your armpits.

Step 4 With each exhale, gently draw your knees toward your armpits, releasing slightly with the inhale.

THINGS TO THINK ABOUT
- Enjoy how your back feels in this pose.

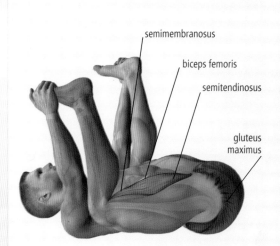

TARGET MUSCLES

semimembranosus

biceps femoris

semitendinosus

gluteus maximus

GLUTES AND HAMSTRINGS

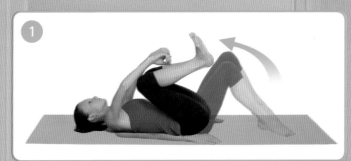

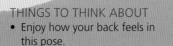

Downward Dog
Adho Mukha Svanasana

The Downward Dog is one of the main poses practiced in yoga. It develops both strength and flexibility. When first starting, you may only be able to hold it for a few breaths, but try to increase that over time. It may look simple, but a lot is happening. This pose is both a forward bend and an inversion. Without kicking up into a handstand, the Downward Dog is a great introduction to the benefits of inversions.

CAUTIONS
- If you have a heart condition, refrain from performing this movement.

THINGS TO THINK ABOUT
- Stretch from your hands to your hips, to create length in your spine.

Step 1 Starting from the Table pose, move your arms forward about the length of one hand. Your hands should be shouder-width apart, fingers spread. Externally rotate your upper arms. With your feet hip-width apart, tuck your toes under. Press into your hands and feet as you begin to straighten your legs.

Step 2 Continue to straighten your legs (your heels do not have to touch the mat).

Step 3 With your feet parallel, activate the muscles in your legs, and lift and spread your buttocks bones.

Step 4 Energize your arms and stretch from your armpits to your hips. On your next exhalation, lower your knees to the floor.

TARGET MUSCLES

gluteus maximus

erector spinae

semitendinosus

biceps femoris

latissimus dorsi

semimembranosus

gastrocnemius

pectoralis major

pectoralis minor

ARMS AND BACK

2

MODIFICATION

If the back of your legs are tight, lift your heels away from the floor.

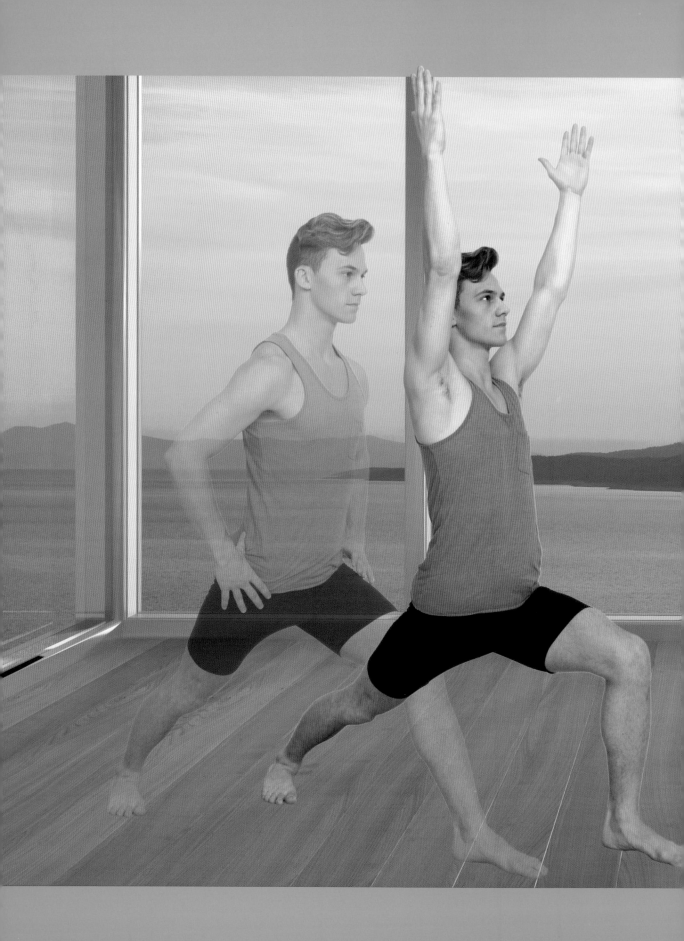

Standing and Balancing Poses

This group of poses is a foundational part of any yogi's practice, beginner through experienced. These poses develop concentration, coordination, balance, poise, strength, and groundedness. They stabilize and strengthen the leg and hip joints, back, shoulders, and neck. These poses teach your legs and arms to stretch, which enables the spine to lengthen and the chest to broaden. Standing and balancing poses invigorate the nervous system. This demands increased circulation and respiration, resulting in an increase in body heat, full-body energy, confidence, stability, and endurance.

Mountain Pose
Tadasana

The Mountain pose may look like "just standing," but the movement in this pose—and the attention required—is intended to practice full-body focus. Continue to move through your body, reminding yourself to engage the appropriate muscles to support the pose. Working well in this pose takes great energy and stamina.

Step 1 Standing with your feet together or slightly apart for more stability, press into all four corners of your feet. Lift and spread your toes back down onto the mat.

Step 2 Activate your legs, and draw the muscles of your thighs up and toward your midline.

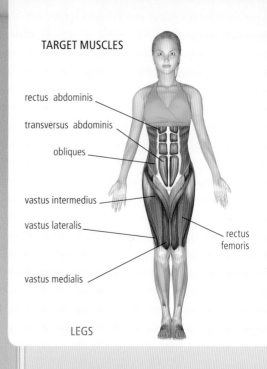

TARGET MUSCLES

rectus abdominis

transversus abdominis

obliques

vastus intermedius

vastus lateralis

rectus femoris

vastus medialis

LEGS

Step 3 To neutralize the pelvis, lengthen your tailbone toward your heels and gently energize your abdominal muscles.

Step 4 Lift your ribs up to elongate your spine. Lift your breastbone, being conscious not to sway your back.

Step 5 Activate the muscles of your arms. Palms facing forward, stretch down through your fingertips, draw your upper arms back, and balance your head over your tailbone. Keep your chest open and turn your palms to face your body.

THINGS TO THINK ABOUT
- Although it looks like not much is happening, many muscles are engaged when this pose is done with intention.

Upward Salute
Urdhva Hastasana

This is another pose that, when done well, is more challenging than it looks. Take your Mountain pose and lift your arms overhead. Use the appropriate muscles in this pose to keep the "shape," but notice if you are engaging muscles that are not needed in this pose. Be aware of the top of shoulders, neck, and jaw. Can you relax these areas and still hold the pose?

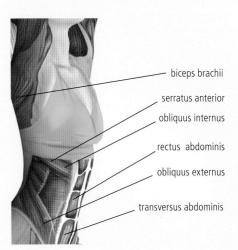

TARGET MUSCLES

biceps brachii
serratus anterior
obliquus internus
rectus abdominis
obliquus externus
transversus abdominis

ABDOMINALS

Step 1 From the Mountain pose, stretch through the fingertips.

Step 2 Externally rotate your arms and lift them over your head, with palms facing each other. Keep your arms straight and parallel. Again, press into your feet and stretch up through your fingertips.

THINGS TO THINK ABOUT
• Holding this pose with intention is harder than it seems.

MODIFICATION

If your shoulders are tight, your arms can be in a wider "V."

Chair Pose
Utkatasana

The Chair pose teaches your body how to hinge at the ankles, knees, and hips. This pose requires full-body strength to hold it. You'll definitely know where your quads are after this! At first, you may only hold it for a few breaths; over time, try to extend the pose, building leg and upper-body strength.

Step 1 Stand in the Mountain pose with your feet together.

Step 2 As you exhale, slowly bend your ankles, knees, and hips as you "sit" down into the pose.

Step 3 Inhale and externally rotate your arms, lifting them out to the side and up, arms parallel, palms facing each other.

Step 4 Tilt your tailbone down so that your back is not overly arched. Lift the side ribs and chest, and keep the back of your neck long. After three or four breaths, on the inhale press into your feet and lift back up into the Mountain pose. Exhale to release your arms out and down to your sides.

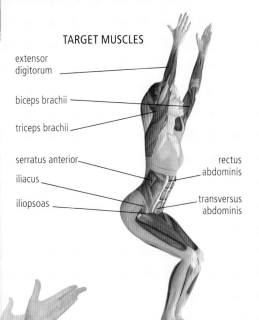

TARGET MUSCLES

- extensor digitorum
- biceps brachii
- triceps brachii
- serratus anterior
- iliacus
- iliopsoas
- rectus abdominis
- transversus abdominis

QUADRICEPS

MODIFICATION

If there is too much tension on your shoulders or neck, your hands can be wider, on your hips or in prayer.

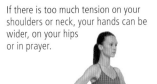

THINGS TO THINK ABOUT

- As you sit your buttocks back and down, drop your tailbone a little and squeeze your legs to your midline.

High Lunge

The High Lunge is a great pose to stretch many of the muscles of the upper thighs and groin. We spend a lot of time in chairs, and the High Lunge is a great pose to counter tightness. At the same time your right side is stretching, your left quad is strengthening. Multitasking at its best!

Step 1 Start standing in the Mountain pose.

Step 2 Exhale as you fold forward into the Chair pose. Bend your knees if you need to so that your hands touch the floor.

Step 3 Step your left foot far enough back so that your front knee is directly over your ankle.

Step 4 Gently rest on your fingertips, gaze forward, and open your chest.

Step 5 Press your back thigh toward the ceiling, and your heel toward the back wall.

Step 6 Step forward into the Chair pose and then into the Mountain pose.

MODIFICATION

If your upper back is rounded, place your hands on blocks to give more room to open your chest.

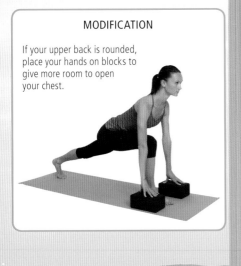

TARGET MUSCLES

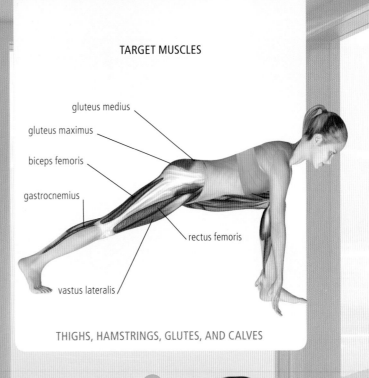

gluteus medius

gluteus maximus

biceps femoris

gastrocnemius

rectus femoris

vastus lateralis

THIGHS, HAMSTRINGS, GLUTES, AND CALVES

THINGS TO THINK ABOUT
• If it is hard to lift your back knee, keep it on the floor at first.

4

Warrior I
Virabhadrasana I

Standing poses are really important to create strength in the legs and open up the groin. The Warrior I is a classic standing pose that increases the energy of the body and creates stamina.

Step 1 Stand at the front edge of your mat.

Step 2 Bend your knees and step your right foot back three feet on an angle, with your toes pointing to the front right corner of the mat.

Step 3 Square your hips to the front and press into the outer edge of your back foot.

MODIFICATION

Place your hands on your hips.

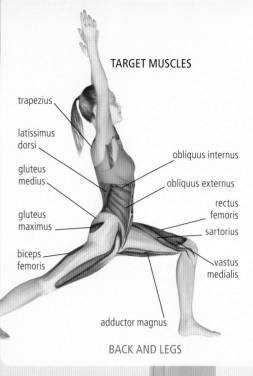

TARGET MUSCLES

trapezius

latissimus dorsi

gluteus medius

gluteus maximus

biceps femoris

obliquus internus

obliquus externus

rectus femoris

sartorius

vastus medialis

adductor magnus

BACK AND LEGS

THINGS TO THINK ABOUT
- Look back at your back foot and make sure it doesn't cross the midline of your mat. Move your foot off to the side.

Step 4 Reach your arms out to your sides, turn your palms up, inhale, and stretch your arms overhead. As you exhale, bend your left knee over your left ankle.

Step 5 Take three breaths.

Step 6 To exit, exhale, put your hands on your hips, and straighten your front leg. Step your back foot up to the front of your mat. Repeat for the other leg.

Warrior II
Virabhadrasana II

The Warrior II pose works different muscles than the Warrior I pose. The challenge is to keep your weight distributed evenly and balance your spine in the center of the pose. With your gaze over the middle finger of your front hand, this pose challenges your spatial awareness to stay aligned when you cannot see.

Step 1 Stand in the middle of your mat, facing the long edge of the mat.

Step 2 Step your feet wide so that when you stretch your arms out to the sides, your heels fall directly under your wrists. Turn your right heel out, and from the top of the left thigh turn your whole left leg and foot out.

MODIFICATION

Place your hands on your hips.

THINGS TO THINK ABOUT
• Keep the top of your shoulders melting down your back, but keep your arms engaged.

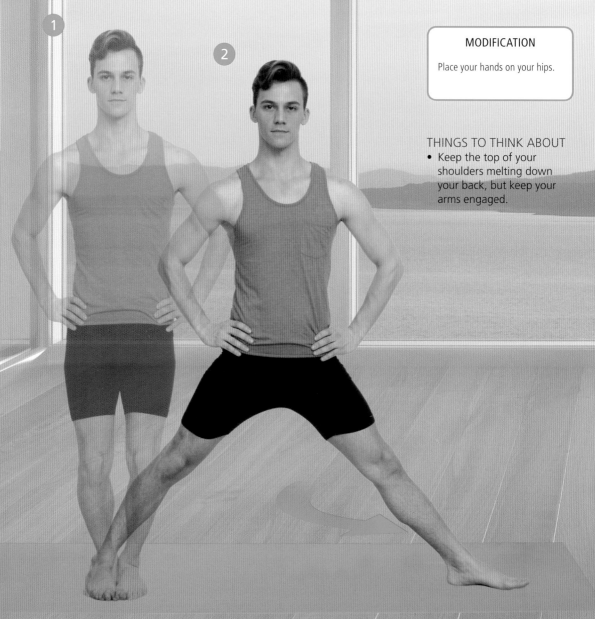

Step 3 Inhale, expand your chest, and lift your arms and stretch through your fingertips.

Step 4 Exhale and bend your left knee over your ankle without passing over your ankle and drawing toward your left.

Step 5 Stretch your right leg by pressing into the outer edge of the right foot.

Step 6 Gaze out over your left fingertips.

Step 7 Keep your arms active, but allow your shoulder to soften.

Step 8 After three breaths, inhale; as you exhale, straighten your left leg, point your toes forward, put your hands on your hips, and hop or walk your feet together.

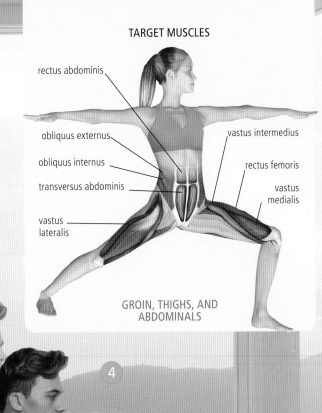

TARGET MUSCLES

rectus abdominis

obliquus externus

obliquus internus

transversus abdominis

vastus lateralis

vastus intermedius

rectus femoris

vastus medialis

GROIN, THIGHS, AND ABDOMINALS

Triangle Pose
Trikonasana

The Triangle is an elegant, powerful pose. Being able to strongly hold this pose and create expansion at the same time is a challenge. Think about your energy concentrated in the center of your torso, and expanding out in five different directions.

THINGS TO THINK ABOUT
- Initially keep your nose in line with your breastbone; if your neck is comfortable, look up at the upraised hand.

Step 1 Stand in the middle of your mat.

Step 2 Step your feet wide so that when you stretch your arms out to the sides, your heels fall directly under your wrists. Turn your right heel out, and from the top of your left thigh turn your whole left leg and foot out.

MODIFICATION

Place your hands on your hips. If you have neck issues, look down. Place your bottom hand on a block.

Step 3 Press into your feet to firm your leg muscles. Inhale, raising your arms out to the side. Expand and lengthen through the spine.

Step 4 Exhale, shift your hips to the right, and hinge at your left hip, bringing your spine over your right leg.

Step 5 Lower your left hand onto your left shin or behind the right shin on the mat or a block and stretch your right arm up.

Step 6 Lean back and open your chest; turn your breastbone toward the sky.

Step 7 After three breaths, inhale and then exhale; press into your feet, pull your belly button to your spine, and lift your torso back to the center. Turn your toes forward and release your arms down. Repeat for the other side.

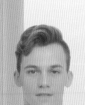

TARGET MUSCLES

obliquus externus

tensor fasciae latae

vastus lateralis

HAMSTRINGS AND GROIN

Extended Side Angle
Utthita Parsvakonasana

The Extended Side Angle pose is a combination of the Warrior II and Triangle poses, and takes your flexibility and strength to a new level. Hold this pose for three breaths, and try to increase that over time. Challenge yourself to keep your front knee bent, transitioning through Warrior II, to exit the pose. Move gracefully, with a sense of purpose.

Step 1 Stand in the middle of your mat. Step your feet wide so that when you stretch your arms out to the sides, your heels fall under your wrists.

Step 2 Turn your right heel out. From the top of your left thigh, turn your whole left leg and foot out.

Step 3 Inhale with your arms out to the side. Expand and lengthen through your spine, exhale, and bend your left knee over your ankle, as your knee presses toward the outer edge of your foot.

THINGS TO THINK ABOUT
- Watch your front knee: keep it in line with your ankle.
- Activate your legs, and keep pressing through the back leg.

TARGET MUSCLES

biceps
brachii

sartorius

semimembranosus

semitendinosus

rectus femoris

ABDOMINALS AND HAMSTRINGS

Step 6 Draw your shoulder blades together on your back to open your chest.

Step 7 After three breaths, inhale, press into your feet, and engage your legs. As you exhale, lift your torso back up into the Warrior II pose. Straighten your left leg, point your toes forward, put your hands on your hips, and hop or walk your feet together.

4

Step 4 Place your left forearm on your left thigh, trying to keep your torso straight. Stretch your right arm over your right leg, turn your palm up, and lift it up over your ear.

Step 5 Stretch from the outer edge of the right foot to your right fingertips.

MODIFICATION

Place your bottom hand on your thigh or on a block.

Intense Side Stretch
Parsvottanasana

The shape of this pose and its name don't seem to correspond. In this pose you will fully engage your legs, and the obvious stretch is at the back of your front leg (hamstring). Once this is established, the focus is on extending out through the top of your head, bringing a lengthening of the two sides of your body, hence the name. Think about moving your shoulders away from your hips to create more space for your rib cage.

Step 1 From the Mountain pose, step your right foot back three feet.

Step 2 Turn your back foot at an angle and press into the outer edge.

Step 3 Place your hands on your hips, elbows back. Square and level your hips. Press into your feet, pull up through your legs, and inhale as you lift your breastbone.

Step 4 Exhale and slowly extend your spine over your left leg, keeping your hips level and squared as you slowly fold forward, keeping your back flat.

Step 5 Keep your hands on your hips and draw your shoulder blades toward each other as you lengthen.

Step 6 Rest your fingertips on the floor or on blocks.

Step 7 Continue to square your hips and firm your leg muscles.

Step 8 After three breaths, to come out, reengage your legs, draw your belly button in, put your hands on your hips with your elbows back, and inhale.

Step 9 Exhale, pressing into your feet and lifting your torso back up.

Step 10 Step forward into the Mountain pose.

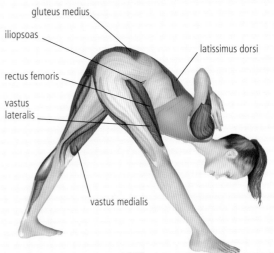

TARGET MUSCLES

gluteus medius

iliopsoas

latissimus dorsi

rectus femoris

vastus lateralis

vastus medialis

LEGS

MODIFICATION

Place your hands on blocks.

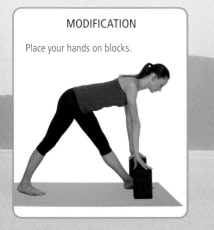

THINGS TO THINK ABOUT
* This pose looks easy, but is quite challenging.

6

Revolved Triangle
Parivrtta Trikonasana

The Revolved Triangle pose is a very challenging pose. This pose is a standing pose, forward bend, and twist all rolled into one. Try to keep your hips level and twist mainly from your middle to upper spine. This may cause you to be unbalanced, so work into this pose slowly and with full awareness. Use the wall to support your back if needed.

Step 1 From the Mountain pose, step your left foot back 3 feet. Place your foot at an angle and press into the outer edge. Place your hands on your hips, elbows back. Square and level your hips. Press into your feet, pull up through your legs, and inhale as you lift your breastbone.

Step 2 Exhale and slowly extend your spine over your right leg. Keep your hips level and squared as you slowly fold forward with a flat back.

Step 3 Revolve over your front leg, bring your left hand to your right shin (or to the floor or a block on the outside of your right leg, depending on ability).

Step 4 Try to square off the hips. (Your left hip will likely need to lower toward the floor.)

1

MODIFICATION

Place your bottom hand on a block or inside of your foot, with your top hand on your hip. If you have neck issues, look forward rather than up.

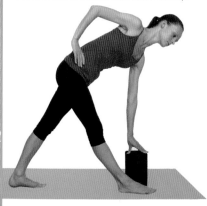

Step 5 If you have no discomfort in your neck, your gaze can go to the ceiling as you draw your shoulder blades together on your back, opening your chest. Lift your right arm up, palm facing to your right.

Step 6 After three breaths, to come out, reengage your legs, draw your belly button in, put your hands on your hips, with your elbows back, and inhale.

Step 7 Exhale, press into your feet, and lift your torso back up.

Step 8 Step forward into the Mountain pose.

CAUTIONS
- If you have any problems with your lower back or sacrum, please refrain from doing this pose.

THINGS TO THINK ABOUT
- This pose is difficult. It is a combination of a standing pose, forward bend, and twist. It may take years to feel comfortable in it!

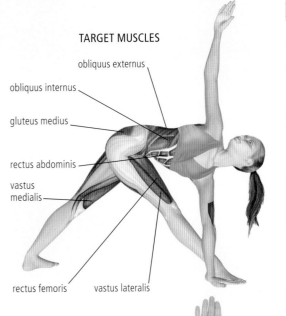

TARGET MUSCLES

obliquus externus

obliquus internus

gluteus medius

rectus abdominis

vastus medialis

rectus femoris

vastus lateralis

ABDOMINALS AND THIGHS

Tree Pose
Vrksasana

The Tree pose is a great introduction to balancing poses. With so many levels within the pose, it is accessible to everyone. To balance, you must draw upon the strength of the feet, legs, and core. Play with arm variations to see how they change the pose. For an added challenge, try closing your eyes.

Step 1 Stand in the Mountain pose. Find a focus point (drishti).

Step 2 Activate your right, standing leg. Keep your hip bones level and pointed forward. Turn your left knee out and draw your left foot high into your groin or to the side of your shin, above your knee. Pressing your foot and thigh together strongly, press your left knee back, keeping your hips stable.

Step 3 Energize your arms by your side, turn your palms out, and stretch them out to the side and overhead, with your hands shoulder-width apart. Lengthen your tailbone down and lift up through your torso. Stretch down through your leg and up through your fingertips.

Step 4 After three breaths, release your arms out and down to the sides. Release your left leg and foot back to the floor, into the Mountain pose.

THINGS TO THINK ABOUT
- Place your hands on your hips and notice if your hip points are level.

MODIFICATIONS

To make the pose easier, you can use a kickstand, block, and wall for support; you could also place your hands on your hips.

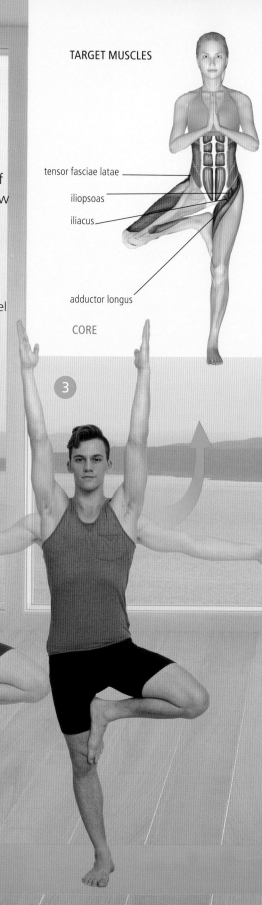

TARGET MUSCLES

tensor fasciae latae

iliopsoas

iliacus

adductor longus

CORE

Eagle Pose
Garudasana

At first, the Eagle pose might feel like a jumble of arms and legs. It is almost like rubbing your stomach and patting your head. In this pose your arms and legs do the opposite on each side. But if that is too confusing, don't worry, just make sure you do the opposite when you change sides! Focus on squeezing to your midline, like you are wringing out a sponge.

Step 1 Start in the Mountain pose. Place your hands on your hips. Extend your left leg to the side and point your toes. Bring your weight to your right leg and bend your right knee. Lift your left leg and wrap it over your right thigh. Depending on flexibility, hook your left foot behind your right ankle. Rebalance and square your hip points.

Step 2 Lift your arms out to the side, with your elbows bent and fingertips pointing to the ceiling. Cross your left arm under your right, bend your elbows, continue to wrap your forearms, and bring your palms together, with your fingertips pointing straight up, and your elbows at shoulder height.

Step 3 Keep your knees bent and your hips folded and square to the front.

Step 4 After three breaths, on the inhale, release your arms and leg out to the sides; on the exhale, come back to the Mountain pose.

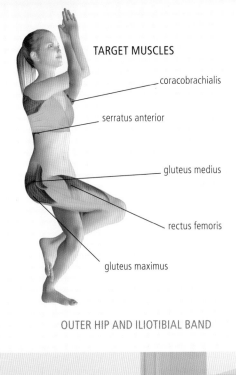

TARGET MUSCLES

coracobrachialis

serratus anterior

gluteus medius

rectus femoris

gluteus maximus

OUTER HIP AND ILIOTIBIAL BAND

CAUTIONS
- Keep your standing knee in line with your ankle.

THINGS TO THINK ABOUT
- If you feel any discomfort in your knees, unwrap.

1

2

MODIFICATIONS

You can place a block under your foot. Only wrap either your arms or your legs.

King Dancer
Natarajasana

The King Dancer is another pose that you can work toward incrementally, making it accessible for all levels. Besides the flexibility that is needed in the back leg, hip, shoulder, and back, you need to balance on one foot! You may wobble—go with it. And realize that the experience of "trying to balance" is what builds the strength to eventually balance and hold the pose. Embrace the wobbles!

Step 1 Stand in the Mountain pose. Shift your weight to the left foot and leg. Bend your right knee, with your heel toward your buttock, and take ahold of the outside of your right ankle with your right hand.

MODIFICATION

If you have balance issues, place your top hand on a wall for support, or just stretch up and don't fold forward.

THINGS TO THINK ABOUT
- Stretch up through your arm and back through your leg before bending back.

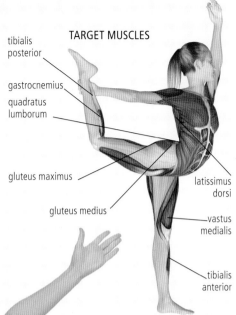

TARGET MUSCLES

tibialis posterior

gastrocnemius

quadratus lumborum

gluteus maximus

gluteus medius

latissimus dorsi

vastus medialis

tibialis anterior

PSOAS, HAMSTRINGS, AND ILIOPSOAS

Step 2 Lift your left arm up, palm facing forward. Realign your hips and knees. Lengthen your tailbone down.

Step 3 Continue to stretch up out of your left side and left hand, and press your right foot back into your right hand until you feel a mild stretch in the front of your right thigh.

Step 4 Hinge forward at the hips, keeping your hips level and square.

Step 5 After three breaths, with awareness, lift back to vertical, release your foot, lower your arm, and stand in the Mountain pose.

Half Moon
Ardha Chandrasana

As with all balancing poses, the Half Moon requires focus and determination, but once in the pose, there is a sense of expansion and freedom. At first, keep your gaze down. Make sure your toes point directly forward and line up with your knee. Keep your back leg energized and press the sole of your back foot behind you.

Step 1 Start in the Warrior II pose, and place your right hand on your hip.

Step 2 Gaze down at your front foot. Shift your weight onto your front foot and shorten your stance as you reach your right hand toward the floor, out beyond your front foot.

Step 3 Begin to straighten your front leg as you start to lift your back leg upward.

Step 4 Place your left hand under your shoulder. Gaze at your fingertips.

Step 5 Open your left hip so it is stacked on top of your right hip. Your top hand can be on your hip or extended, fingertips to the ceiling.

Step 6 To exit the pose, bend your front knee, gracefully and with control, stepping your left foot back into the Warrior II pose.

TARGET MUSCLES

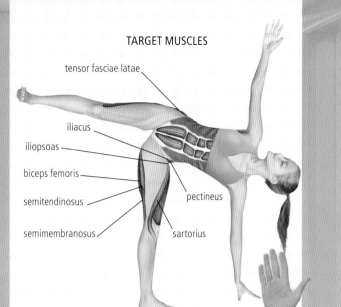

tensor fasciae latae

iliacus

iliopsoas

biceps femoris

semitendinosus

semimembranosus

pectineus

sartorius

GROIN

MODIFICATIONS

Place one hand on a block, and the other on your hip. If you have neck pain, look down.

THINGS TO THINK ABOUT
- If you have difficulty balancing, practice this pose next to a wall. Place your back to the wall and use the wall as support.
- As you hone your balance, challenge yourself to shift your gaze to the ceiling.
- You can simplify the pose by resting your hand on a block.

5

Warrior III
Virabhadrasana III

Practicing balance poses can be humbling. The same pose can change dramatically from day to day. The Warrior III gets more challenging as you pivot toward full expression of the pose. Remember that you can always start off small. Keep your hands on your hips and only raise your rear leg a few inches at first. You are still in the pose.

THINGS TO THINK ABOUT
- Stretch back through the flexed foot and forward through the top of your head.
- Think "extension" instead of "folding forward."

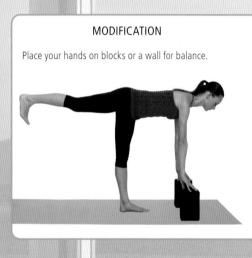

MODIFICATION

Place your hands on blocks or a wall for balance.

Step 1 Stand in the Mountain pose. Choose an arm position: hands on hips, hands in prayer, or hands over head. Engage your legs, shifting your weight onto your left foot and leg.

1

TARGET MUSCLES

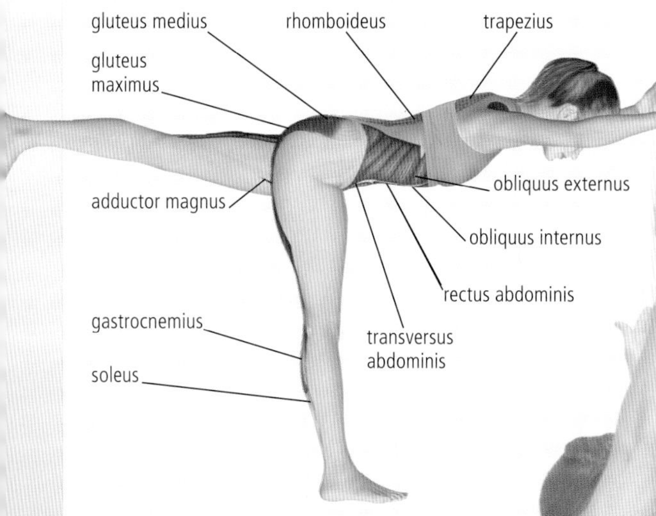

gluteus medius
rhomboideus
trapezius
gluteus maximus
adductor magnus
obliquus externus
obliquus internus
rectus abdominis
gastrocnemius
transversus abdominis
soleus

LEGS

Step 2 Draw your belly button to your spine. Hinge forward at your hip, lifting your right leg behind you.

Step 3 Flex your back foot and press out through your heel, keeping your head in line with the rest of your spine.

Step 4 Hold for 3 breaths.

Step 5 Inhale and hinge back to a standing position.

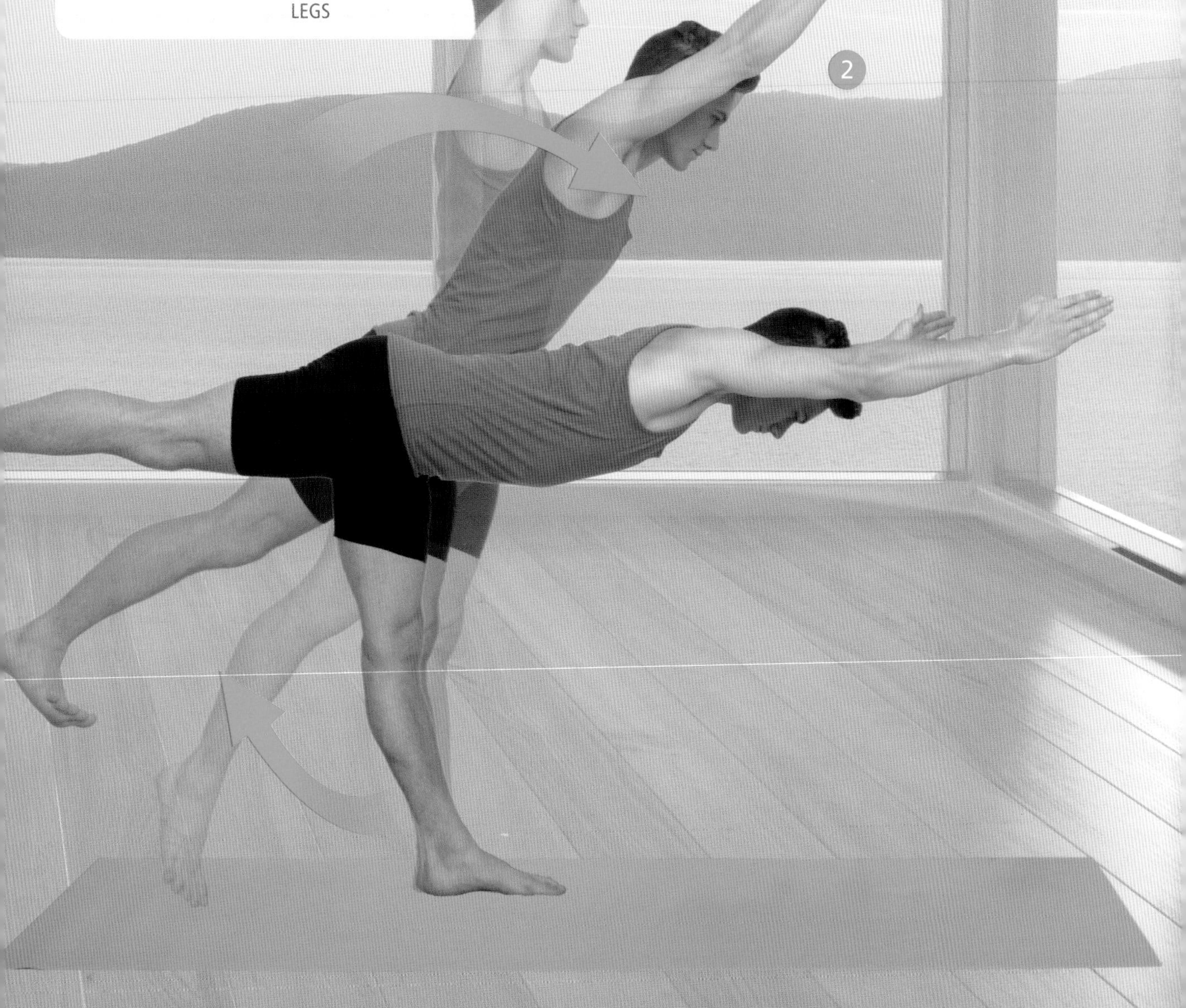

2

Extended Hand to Big Toe
Utthita Hasta Padangusthasana

All balancing poses demand a high level of focus and concentration, but this is one of the more challenging ones. The balance in this pose is not static: the conscious effort of entering into this pose, moving through it, and returning to where you started develops a great amount of focus. A fully engaged mind and body are needed to access the stamina, strength, flexibility, and balance to be in this pose—or out you fall!

Step 1 Stand in the Mountain pose. Find a focus point. Shift your weight to your right foot, grounding all four corners of your foot. Place your right hand on your hip.

Step 2 Bend your left leg, with your knee lifted up toward your chest. Keeping the hips square, and the standing leg straight, begin to straighten the left leg in front of you.

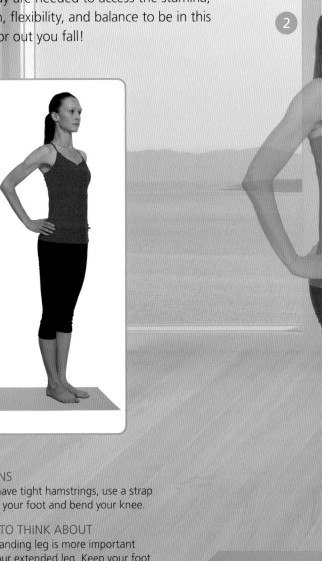

CAUTIONS
• If you have tight hamstrings, use a strap to hold your foot and bend your knee.

THINGS TO THINK ABOUT
• Your standing leg is more important than your extended leg. Keep your foot pointing forward, with your leg straight and engaged. The other leg position will come with practice.

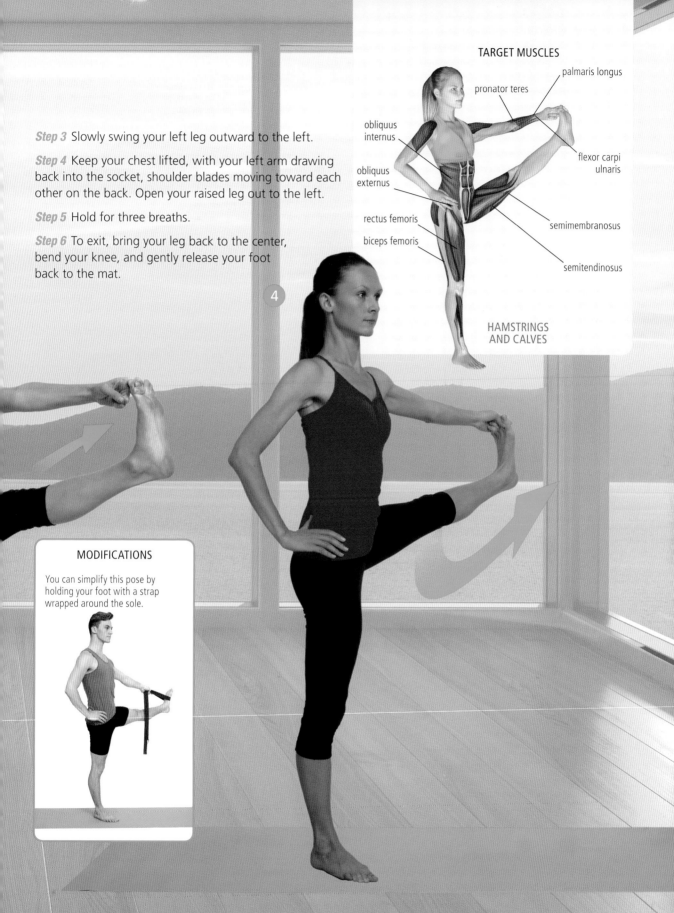

Step 3 Slowly swing your left leg outward to the left.

Step 4 Keep your chest lifted, with your left arm drawing back into the socket, shoulder blades moving toward each other on the back. Open your raised leg out to the left.

Step 5 Hold for three breaths.

Step 6 To exit, bring your leg back to the center, bend your knee, and gently release your foot back to the mat.

TARGET MUSCLES

palmaris longus

pronator teres

obliquus internus

flexor carpi ulnaris

obliquus externus

rectus femoris

biceps femoris

semimembranosus

semitendinosus

HAMSTRINGS AND CALVES

MODIFICATIONS

You can simplify this pose by holding your foot with a strap wrapped around the sole.

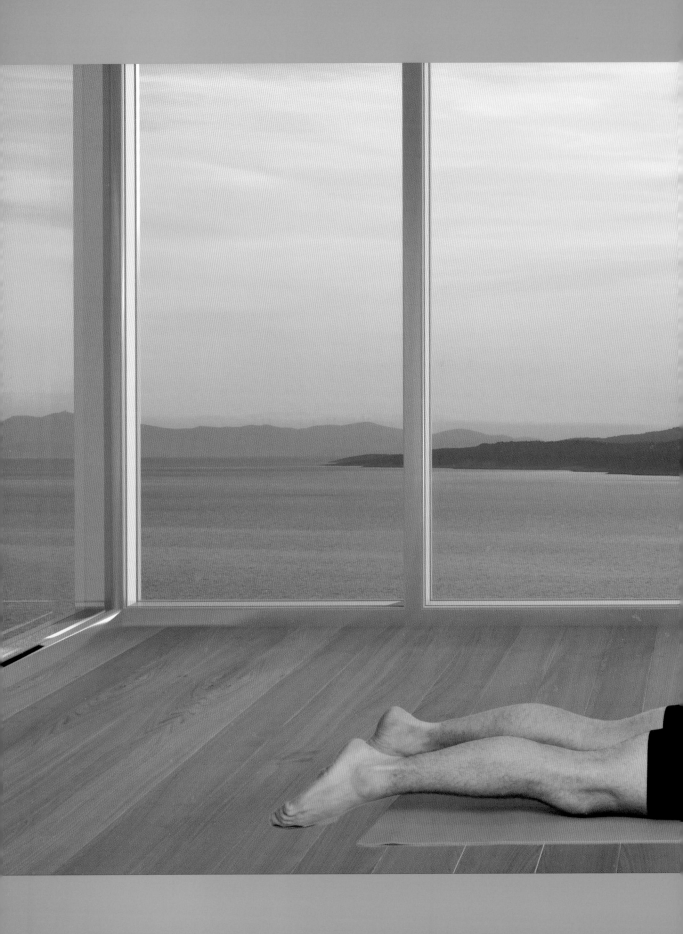

Back Bends

So many of our daily activities are centered around sitting. Back bends are incredibly important to counter the forward folding of the spine and hunching of the upper back as we sit in chairs and cars. Back bends are key to strengthening the arms, shoulders, and back muscles. As the back muscles contract, the chest expands, facilitating deeper breathing, improvement of blood circulation, and increased body heat. Back bends decongest and invigorate the nervous system.

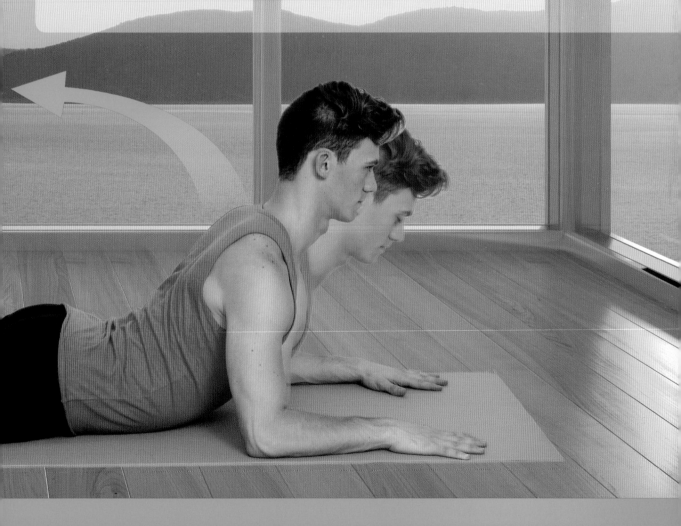

Sphinx Pose

Remember when you were a teenager and you watched TV lying on the floor, propped up on your elbows? Even if you didn't realize at the time, this position was much healthier than slouching on a sofa. The Sphinx pose engages the muscles of the upper back and opens the chest, reversing the effects of driving a car or sitting in front of the computer for hours on end.

Step 1 Lie stretched out on your stomach.

Step 2 Prop yourself up on your elbows. Bring your elbows under your shoulders, forearms parallel with your elbows and wrists shoulder-width apart, fingers spread.

Step 3 With your feet roughly hip-width apart, stretch back through your toes.

Step 4 Draw your belly button to your spine, and press your pubic bone into the floor, lengthening your tailbone.

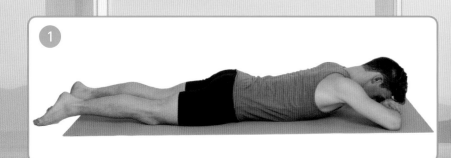

CAUTIONS
• Avoid or modify this pose if you have lower-back pain.

THINGS TO THINK ABOUT
• This is a simple back bend, but it is very beneficial!

Step 5 Draw your shoulder blades together, and lift your breastbone forward and up.

Step 6 Further open the chest by isometrically pulling your hands toward your chest.

Step 7 After three breaths, with awareness, lower yourself, cross your arms to make a pillow, turn your cheek to the side, and rest.

MODIFICATION

If this pose doesn't feel appropriate on your lower back, try lowering your chest by widening your elbows.

TARGET MUSCLES

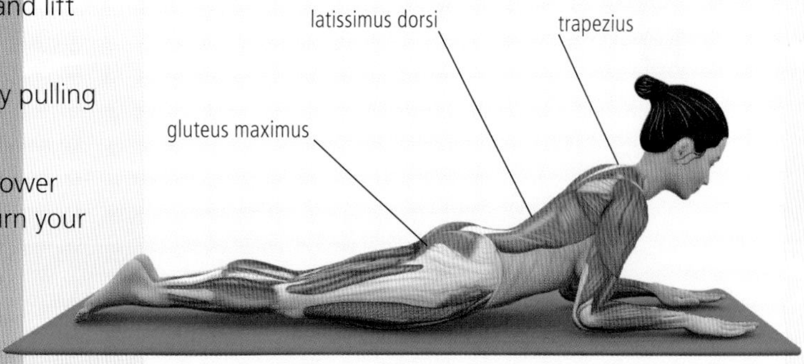

latissimus dorsi

trapezius

gluteus maximus

UPPER BACK

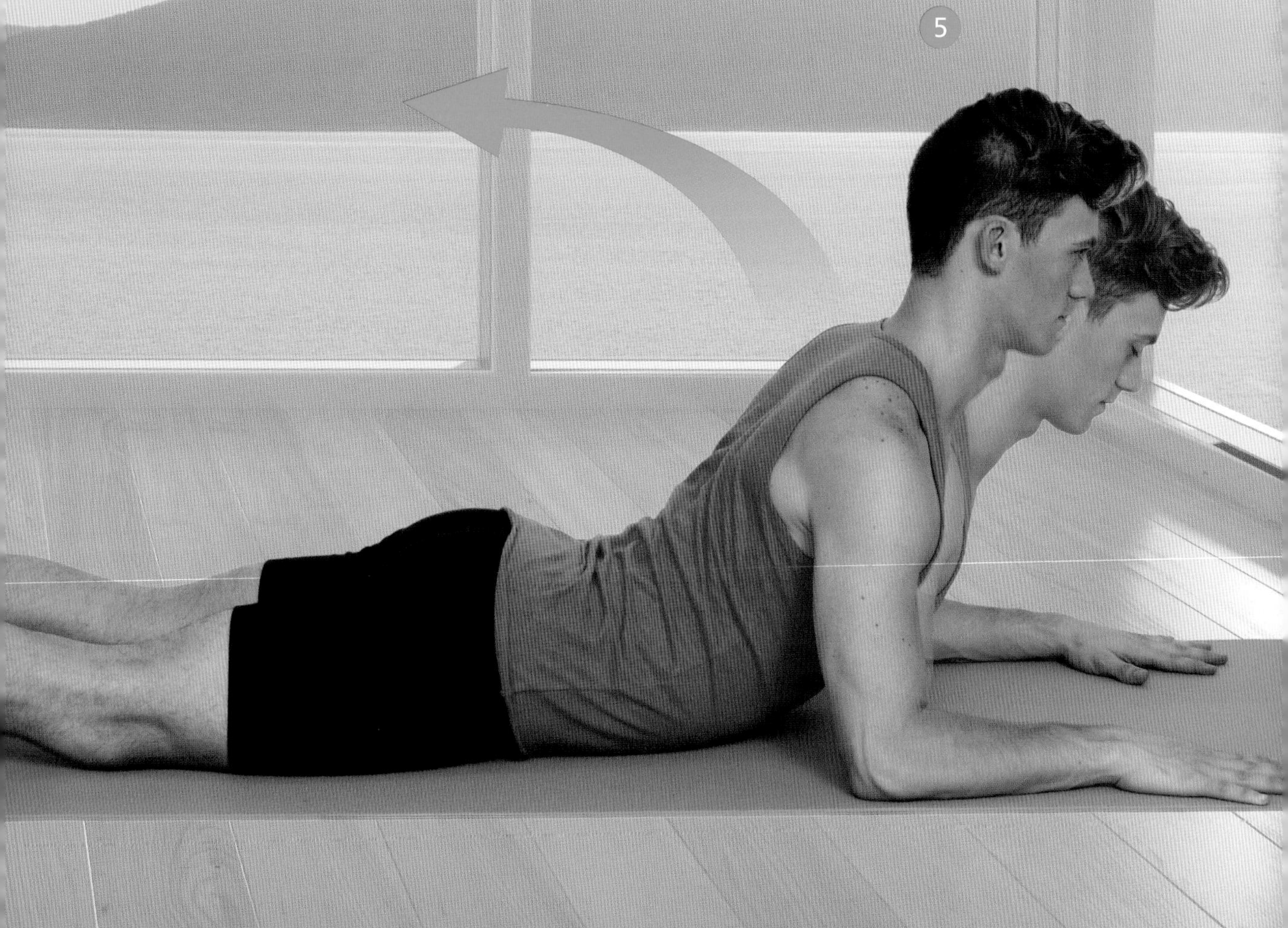

5

Cobra Pose
Bhujangasana

Even if the Upward Dog (page 66) and more advanced back bends are in your routine, don't skip this pose. The Cobra pose is so important in the development of your flexibility. Always start off with the simple back bends, and eventually move toward more difficult poses. Spend time in the Cobra pose working the muscles of your upper back to open your chest. To check if you are accessing those muscles, try taking some of the weight out of your hands and see if you can still hold the pose.

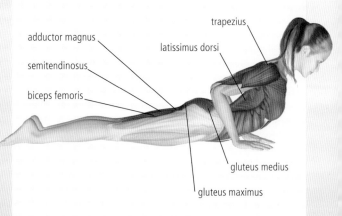

TARGET MUSCLES

adductor magnus
semitendinosus
biceps femoris
trapezius
latissimus dorsi
gluteus medius
gluteus maximus

CORE AND HAMSTRINGS

Step 1 Lie on your stomach, forehead to the floor.

Step 2 Place your hands alongside your chest, fingers pointing forward, elbows pointing to the ceiling.

Step 3 With your legs about one foot apart, internally rotate the thighs and stretch back through your toes.

Step 4 Pull your hands back so the heels of the palms are next to your lower ribs.

Step 5 Draw your elbows to your midline and lift the front of your shoulders away from the floor.

Step 6 Draw your belly button to your spine, and press your pubic bone into the floor, lengthening your tailbone.

Step 7 Lift your head in line with your spine. Curl your head, neck, and chest up and away from the floor.

Step 8 Lengthen from the crown of your head to your toes.

Step 9 After three breaths, slowly and with awareness, lower yourself to the floor, arms down by your side, palms up, cheek to the side, and rest.

CAUTIONS
• Avoid or modify this pose if you have lower-back pain.

THINGS TO THINK ABOUT
• Move from the upper back only.

MODIFICATION

If you have back issues, keep the back bend small and low.

1

7

5

Locust Pose
Salabasana

When first practicing this pose, you may feel like you aren't getting too far off the floor. If you try to lift up, you may feel a crunch in the lower back. That means you have gone too far. Try to visualize your back in this pose. Keep a balance between lifting up and extending out through the top of your head and toes. Try closing your eyes, and rather than focusing on how far you are off the floor, tune in to the sensations that are rising up in your body.

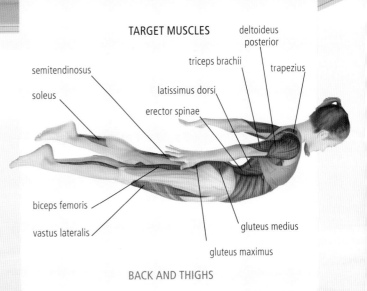

TARGET MUSCLES

semitendinosus
soleus
biceps femoris
vastus lateralis
erector spinae
latissimus dorsi
triceps brachii
deltoideus posterior
trapezius
gluteus medius
gluteus maximus

BACK AND THIGHS

Step 1 Lie on your stomach, forehead to the floor. Bring your arms alongside your body, palms up.

Step 2 With your legs hip-width apart, and your thighs inwardly rotated, stretch back through your toes.

Step 3 Draw your belly button to your spine, and press your pubic bone into the floor, lengthening your tailbone.

Step 4 Draw your arms to your midline and lift the front of your shoulders and arms away from the floor.

Step 5 Keep your neck in line with your spine and stretch your toes away from the top of your head. On your next inhale, lift your head, neck, chest, and legs all at the same time.

Step 6 After three breaths, slowly and with awareness, lower yourself to the floor, arms down by your sides, palms up, cheek to the side, and rest.

CAUTIONS
• Avoid or modify this pose if you have lower-back pain.

THINGS TO THINK ABOUT
• If this is challenging, lift your opposite arm and leg, and rest in between sides.

MODIFICATION

Lift only your arms or legs, rather than both.

Half-Frog Pose
Ardha Bhekasana

The Half-Frog pose develops flexibility in the quads, front of the hips, back, shoulders, and chest. The Half-Frog is considered prep for some of the more advanced poses like the Bow and Wheel, but ironically it takes a good amount of flexibility to actually get into the pose. You may want to stretch your quads out in other ways before beginning this pose. This pose can take years to master, so modifications are always acceptable.

Step 1 Lie on your stomach and move with awareness into the Sphinx pose.

Step 2 Turn your left forearm in parallel to the front edge of the mat.

Step 3 Drawing your belly into your spine, press your pubic bone into the floor, lengthening your tailbone.

Step 4 Bend your right knee and reach back with your right hand for the inside of your right foot. Pull your foot toward your buttock.

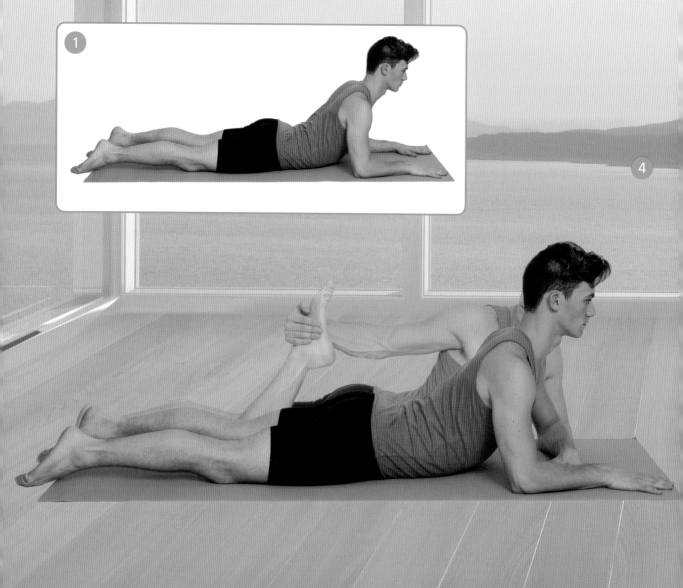

Step 5 Keep your knees parallel and both hips on the floor. Raise your elbow up and face forward.

Step 6 After three breaths, release your foot and rest.

CAUTIONS
* Avoid this pose if you have knee pain. If you have lower-back pain, keep your forehead on the floor, or refrain from doing this pose.

THINGS TO THINK ABOUT
* At first, feel free to let your knee open out to the side, but as the front of your leg stretches, begin to move your knee toward your midline.

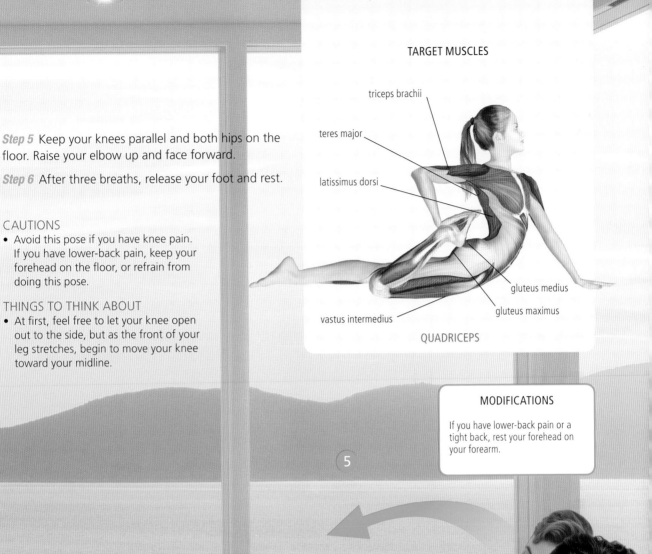

TARGET MUSCLES

triceps brachii

teres major

latissimus dorsi

gluteus medius

gluteus maximus

vastus intermedius

QUADRICEPS

MODIFICATIONS
If you have lower-back pain or a tight back, rest your forehead on your forearm.

5

Bow Pose
Dhanurasana

The Bow pose is a deep back bend. Your body makes the shape of an archer's bow; your arms are the strings. The action of your feet pressing into your hands lifts your shoulders and opens the chest. If you can't reach both ankles, start with one leg at a time and develop the flexibility to eventually work toward both at the same time.

Step 1 Lie on your belly with your arms by your sides, palms up; bring your forehead to the floor. Bend both knees.

Step 2 Reach back for your outer ankles, trying to grab them both at the same time. Draw your shoulder blades into your back.

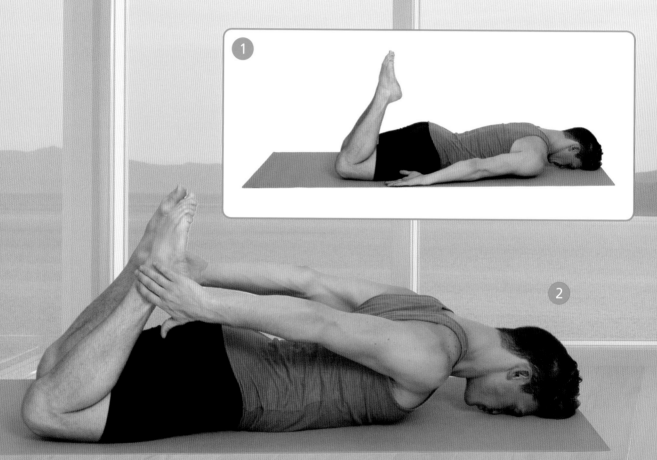

MODIFICATION

Lift up lower if you experience any discomfort.

Step 3 Draw your belly button to your spine and press your pubic bone into the floor, lengthening your tailbone. Press your feet into your hands to lift up. Align your head with your spine. Expand your chest.

Step 4 After three breaths, slowly and with awareness, lower down, release your legs, palms up, cheek to the side, and rest.

CAUTIONS
- If you have discomfort in the knees, widen the knees or avoid this pose.

THINGS TO THINK ABOUT
- Continue to keep your tailbone moving down and your belly button drawing in. Height is not your goal.

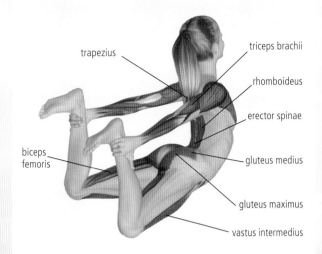

TARGET MUSCLES

trapezius
triceps brachii
rhomboideus
erector spinae
biceps femoris
gluteus medius
gluteus maximus
vastus intermedius

CHEST, THIGHS, AND ARMS

3

Bridge
Setu Bandha Sarvangasana

The Bridge pose is a great beginner pose that most everyone feels good practicing. This pose energizes the body, but also quiets the mind. Breathe deeply and remember to keep your head and neck centered, and your gaze up toward the ceiling, releasing your neck. Notice if you are lifting your hips by clenching your buttocks. Try to release the muscles you don't need.

Step 1 Lie on your back, bend your knees, with the soles of your feet on the mat close to your buttocks, hip-width apart and parallel. Your heels should be under your knees. Have your arms close to your body, palms down.

Step 2 Bend your elbows, fingertips pointing to the ceiling. Press into your upper arms and tuck each shoulder blade under to open your chest.

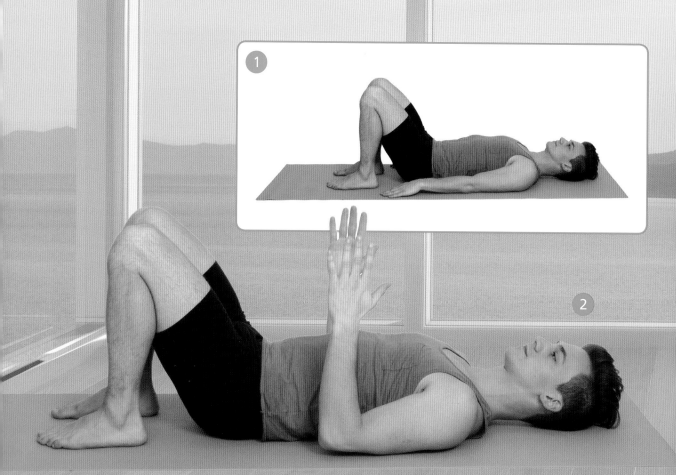

Step 3 Press evenly into the inner and outer edges of your feet. Lengthen your tailbone toward your knees and lift your hips off the floor.

Step 4 Continue to press into your upper arms and open and expand your upper chest. Internally rotate your thighs and relax your buttocks.

Step 5 After three breaths, slowly lower your hips to the floor.

Step 6 Release your arms with your palms up.

CAUTIONS
- Avoid this pose if you have lower-back or neck pain.

THINGS TO THINK ABOUT
- Enjoy this back bend—your ability to breathe deeply in this pose is amazing.

TARGET MUSCLES

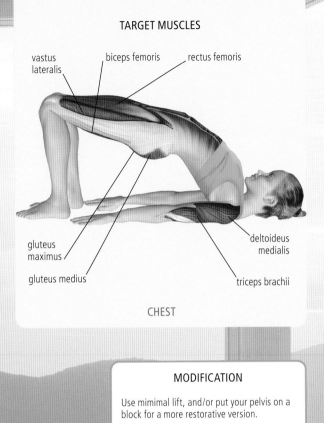

vastus lateralis
biceps femoris
rectus femoris
gluteus maximus
gluteus medius
deltoideus medialis
triceps brachii

CHEST

MODIFICATION

Use mimimal lift, and/or put your pelvis on a block for a more restorative version.

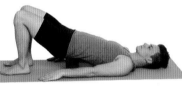

3

Fish Pose
Matsyasana

The Fish pose feels strange because it is! Our bodies never go into this shape. But there is a point; this pose creates a huge chest-opening experience, and the ability to breathe deep feels great. Always monitor your neck in this pose, and release out of this pose consciously. Notice the high level of relaxation that is obtained after this pose.

Step 1 Lie on your back, and stretch long from your head to your feet, elongating your spine.

Step 2 With your arms straight, slide one arm and then the other under your body, palms down.

Step 3 Activate the muscles of your legs and flex your feet at the same time. Inhale, and press your forearms into the ground to prop yourself up. Look at your feet. Tilt your pelvis into a dog tilt. Arch your back and lift your breastbone.

CAUTIONS
• Avoid this pose if you have any neck issues and/or vertigo.

THINGS TO THINK ABOUT
• There aren't many times we stretch the front of throat. Enjoy this stretch, but be mindful as to how your neck feels.

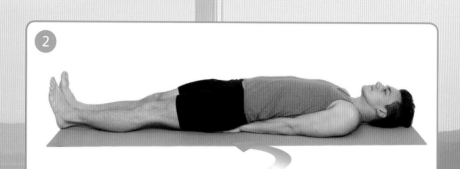

Step 4 Keep the back of your neck long. As you exhale, stretch your throat and rest the top of your head on the ground so the crown of your head rests on the mat.

Step 5 Take three deep breaths, then open your chest and your throat.

Step 6 To exit, engage your abdominals and legs, and on the inhale, press into your arms and hands. Tuck your chin toward your chest and exhale. Release to the floor and rest.

Step 7 Alternatively, slide the back of your head onto the floor to release.

TARGET MUSCLES

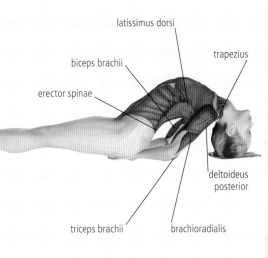

latissimus dorsi

trapezius

biceps brachii

erector spinae

deltoideus posterior

triceps brachii

brachioradialis

BACK

MODIFICATION

Place a block under your shoulder blades and rest the top of your head on a blanket.

4

Upward Dog
Urdhva Mukha Svanasana

This back bend requires a combination of flexibility and strength. You must engage your legs and core to safely practice this pose. If you feel this pose in your lower back, your upper back may be stiff. Work on developing the flexibility in your upper back and the strength in your arms before revisiting this pose.

Step 1 Lie on your stomach, legs stretched long behind you, with the tops of your feet on the floor. Bend your elbows and place your hands, fingers spread and facing forward, at your lower ribs, with your arms hugging your midline.

Step 2 Press your palms into the floor and isometrically draw your hands back, feeling your chest open and your shoulder blades draw together on your back.

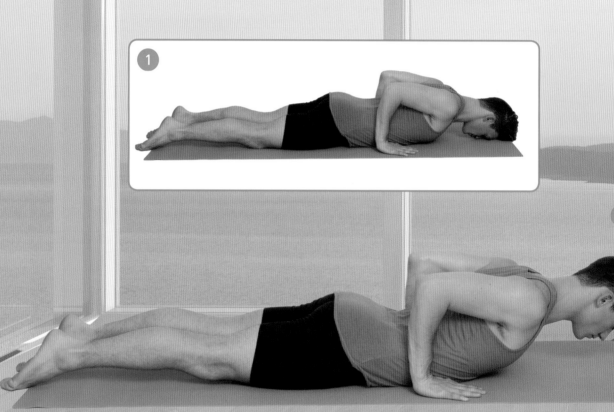

CAUTIONS
• If you feel any discomfort in your lower back, lower toward the floor or refrain from this exercise.

THINGS TO THINK ABOUT
• This is a very strong pose, and the whole body needs to work to hold it.

Step 3 Lengthen your tailbone down, press into the tops of your feet and straighten your arms, lifting your torso and knees off the floor.

Step 4 Keeping your legs engaged, draw your belly button to your spine so your lower back does not sag.

Step 5 Inwardly rotate your thigh and externally rotate your upper arm, turning the outer edge of your elbow forward.

Step 6 Gaze forward or slightly up.

Step 7 Slowly bend your arms to release yourself back down to your belly.

Step 8 Cross your arms and rest your cheek to the side.

MODIFICATIONS

Keep your knees on the floor.

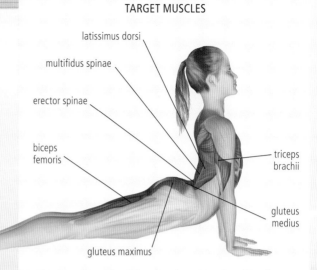

TARGET MUSCLES

latissimus dorsi

multifidus spinae

erector spinae

biceps femoris

triceps brachii

gluteus medius

gluteus maximus

UPPER BODY

Knees-Chest-Chin

Ashtangpranama

This traditional transitional pose is used in sun salutations to move from the Downward Dog to the Cobra or Upward Dog. It takes enormous coordination to move through this pose with ease and grace. If it feels difficult, don't get discouraged—keep practicing. This pose develops arm strength and back flexibility that you will need for more advanced poses like the Upward Dog and Four-Limbed Staff pose (page 120).

Step 1 Start in the Table pose with toes tucked. Move your hands one hand's length forward. Arch your back into a dog tilt.

Step 2 Bend your elbows close to the rib cage, and lower your chest and chin to the floor slightly in front of your hands.

Step 3 Keep your buttocks in the air, with your elbows close to your ribs and pointing to the sky.

Step 4 Press off your toes, sliding through your hands, forward onto your belly.

Step 5 Point your toes, squeeze your elbows to your midline, and arch your upper back to a low Cobra pose.

CAUTIONS
- If you have shoulder injuries, avoid this pose.

THINGS TO THINK ABOUT
- Use this pose to transition.
- Remember to push off your toes to move forward onto your stomach on the mat.

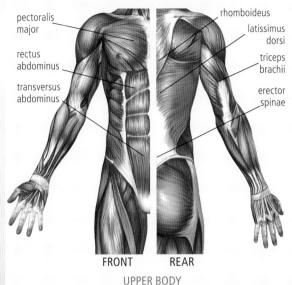

TARGET MUSCLES

pectoralis major
rectus abdominus
transversus abdominus

rhomboideus
latissimus dorsi
triceps brachii
erector spinae

FRONT   REAR

UPPER BODY

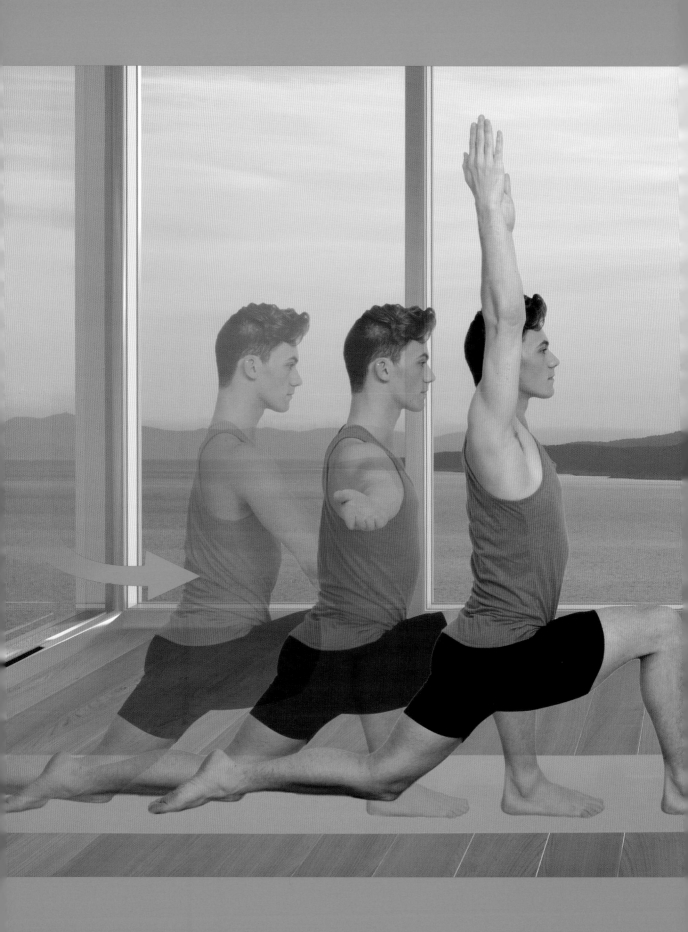

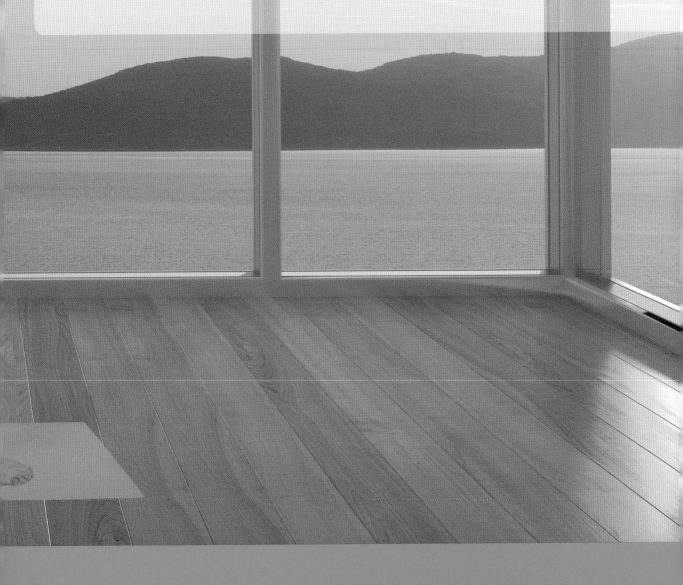

Hip Openers

When we increase flexibility, strength, and balance in the hips, the rest of the body becomes more comfortable. Hip openers stretch the muscles, ligaments, and nerves of the groin, and massage and decongest abdominal organs. This helps improve circulation of bodily fluids between the legs and torso.

Squat Pose
Malasana

In many parts of the world, people spend a lot of time in this pose. Chores and work are done in this pose, families eat, children play, and babies are born. This is an important pose to get back to, and can be done just about anywhere.

Step 1 Stand with your feet hip-width apart (wider if you are tighter), toes pointed outward.

Step 2 Hinge at your hips and knees and sit your buttocks down toward the floor.

Step 3 Place your elbows against the inside of your knees with your hands together. Continue to drop your hips, open your chest, and stretch up through your spine.

Step 4 To release, place your hands on the floor, lift your buttocks up, bring your feet to parallel, and roll up.

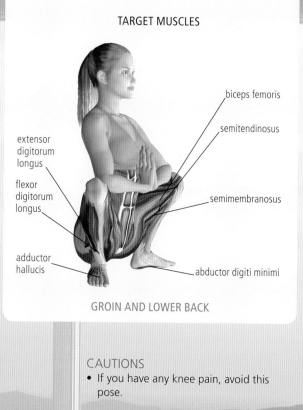

TARGET MUSCLES

biceps femoris

semitendinosus

semimembranosus

abductor digiti minimi

extensor digitorum longus

flexor digitorum longus

adductor hallucis

GROIN AND LOWER BACK

CAUTIONS
• If you have any knee pain, avoid this pose.

THINGS TO THINK ABOUT
• Keep your feet in line with your knees, and continue to drop your tailbone down.

MODIFICATION

If your heels are off the floor, place a rolled blanket underneath them. Place a block under your pelvis for support.

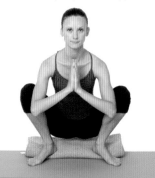

2

3

Gate Pose
Parigasana

The Gate pose is similar to the Triangle, but it takes the legs out of the picture so you can focus on stretching the side body from hip to arm. This is an area that rarely gets stretched. When we finally do start to stretch the sides in this way, the ability to breathe deeper into these spaces increases.

Step 1 Kneel sideways on your mat. Stretch your left leg out to the side, knee and toes facing up.

Step 2 Place your hands on your hips and shift your hips to the left. Release your left hand on your shin for support.

Step 3 Turn your right palm up, stretching your arm up overhead toward your left foot.

Step 4 After three breaths, press into your legs, and lift back up on the inhale. Sit down on your knees.

MODIFICATION

Place your top hand on your hip.

TARGET MUSCLES

obliques

transversus abdominus

adductor longus

OBLIQUES

CAUTIONS
- Pad your bottom knee.

THINGS TO THINK ABOUT
- This pose feels really good. It opens up the side body. We don't get to do that too often in life and in yoga!

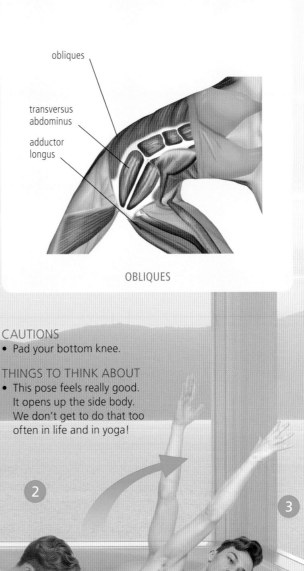

1

2

3

Low Lunge
Anjaneyasana

The Low Lunge stretches the front, back, and inside of the hips and groin. Keeping flexibility in the hips and groin has a ripple effect of releasing lower-back tension. Be very mindful not to sink your hips too far into this pose. Keep your pelvis neutral and your legs engaged.

Step 1 From the Downward Dog, swing your right foot up between your hands, with your ankle in line with your fingertips, and your foot in line with your outer hip.

Step 2 Release your left knee to the mat and untuck your toes. Press your hips forward, keeping your right heel under your knee. Lengthen the stance if necessary to do so.

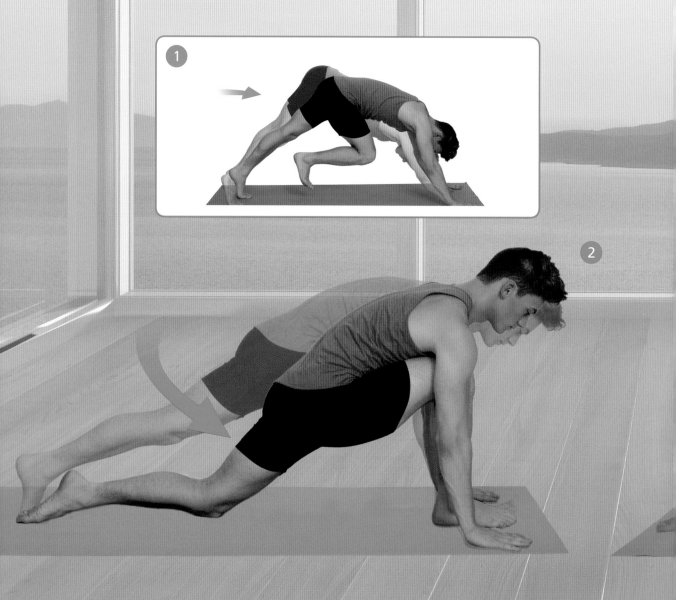

Step 3 Lengthen your tailbone down and lift your pubic bone. Extend your arms up overhead, parallel, palms facing each other. Gaze either forward or up. Hold for three breaths.

Step 4 Release your hands to the mat and press back to the Downward Dog.

THINGS TO THINK ABOUT
• Keep your groin stretched. It will decrease strain in your lower back.

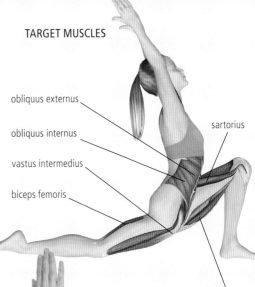

TARGET MUSCLES

obliquus externus

obliquus internus

vastus intermedius

biceps femoris

sartorius

adductor magnus

GROIN

3

MODIFICATION

Place your hands on blocks.

Bound Angle Pose
Baddha Konasana

This pose is found in most yoga classes, from beginner to advanced. The benefits of this pose are so important because the ability to sit on the floor comfortably is only possible with open hips and groin, and strong core and back muscles. Continue to practice this pose no matter how advanced you take your yoga practice.

Step 1 Sitting on a mat, bend your knees and place the soles of your feet together.

Step 2 Adjust your posture until your sitting bones feel grounded.

Step 3 Hold on to your ankles or feet, inhale, and stretch up through the crown of your head to lengthen your spine.

Step 4 As you exhale, fold from your hips, allowing your pubic bone to move toward the floor.

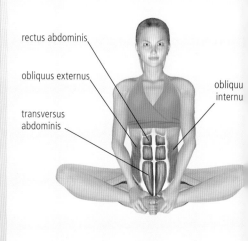

TARGET MUSCLES

rectus abdominis

obliquus externus

obliquu
internu

transversus
abdominis

ABDOMINALS

Step 5 Place your elbows on your knees or in front of your shins. Keep your head in line with your spine and continue to lengthen from your tailbone to the crown of your head.

Step 6 After three breaths, hinge at your hips, lift your torso back up, and release your legs.

THINGS TO THINK ABOUT
- Be in this pose with your back rounded and flat, and feel the difference.
- Engage and relax your feet in this pose, and feel the difference.

1

4

MODIFICATION

If your knees are high, sit on a blanket.

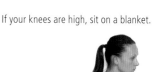

Supine Big Toe Hold
Supta Pada Gustasanana

This pose is an excellent way to stretch the back of the legs, groin, hips, and back. Lying on your back and stretching in this pose is an effective way to get into tight spaces without compromising your back.

Step 1 Lie on your back with your knees bent, feet on the floor. Lift your right leg and put the strap on your foot. Hold the strap with both hands evenly, arms extended fully.

Step 2 Stretch your left leg out on the floor and energize it, internally rotating your upper thigh. Hold for three breaths, and then take the strap in your right hand.

Step 3 Keep your left hip grounded with your left hand, and open your right leg out to the right, hovering above the floor. Keep both legs really active.

Step 4 Draw your right leg into the socket and lift it up to neutral. Switch hands on the strap. Extend your right arm out for stability.

Step 5 Move your right leg across your midline to the left.

Step 6 Lower your leg and hover it above the floor, allowing the bottom foot to roll toward the outside. Keep both legs active and your right shoulder on the floor.

Step 7 After three breaths, ground your right arm and shoulder, draw your belly button to your spine, and lift your leg back up to neutral.

Step 8 Hold the strap with both hands and continue to stretch the back of your leg.

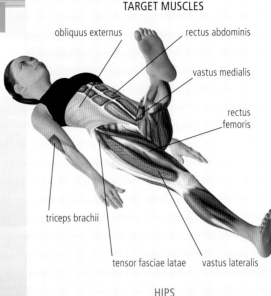

TARGET MUSCLES

obliquus externus

rectus abdominis

vastus medialis

rectus femoris

triceps brachii

tensor fasciae latae

vastus lateralis

HIPS

CAUTIONS
• If you have any lower-back discomfort, avoid this pose. Bend your knee if needed.

THINGS TO THINK ABOUT
• This pose is great for stretching the legs and hips without getting the back too involved. If you have back issues, this pose is a safe way to get the stretch. Use a strap and make the movements smaller.

Cow Face
Gomukhasana

Doing the Cow Face pose, you will quickly learn that our bodies are not perfectly symmetrical. You may be able to get into the pose with your left leg on top, but when you try on the other side, there is a huge gap between your knees. Similarly, your fingers may clasp easily on one side, while you have to use a belt for the other side. Rather than get frustrated, use the props you need to support you, so you can slowly open the tighter spaces.

Step 1 Sit on a mat. Slide your right foot under your left knee and place your right foot outside your left hip, with the outer edge of your foot on the mat.

Step 2 Bring your left leg and foot over your right knee and place it next to your right outer hip. Flex both feet. Stack your knees.

Step 3 Take your fingertips behind your buttocks and stretch up through your spine and chest.

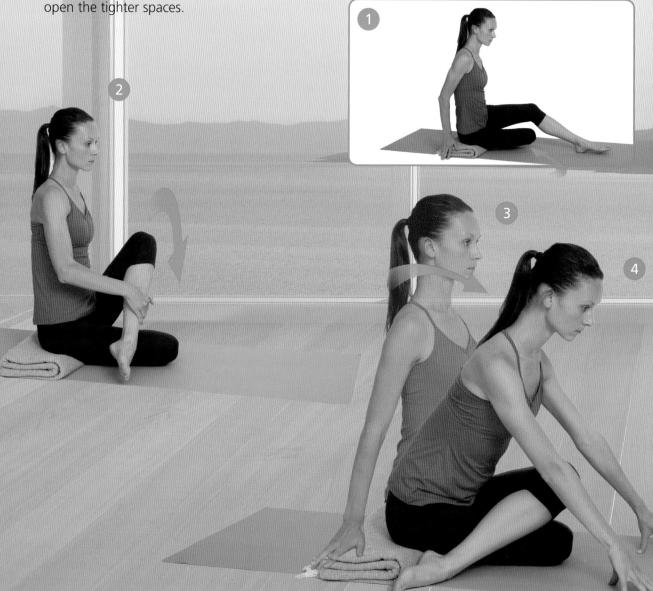

Step 4 For further hip opening, fold forward over the knees.

Step 5 Stretch your left arm out to the side and internally rotate your arm. Bend your elbow and bring your arm behind your back so the back of your hand rests on your back, with your fingers stretching up toward your head.

Step 6 Take your right arm, stretch it out to the side, palm facing the ceiling. Lift your arm up to the ear, and bend your elbow, fingers pointing down.

Step 7 Try to hook your fingers.

Step 8 Keep lifting your right elbow as you draw your left elbow behind you.

Step 9 If you feel comfortable, begin to fold forward over your knees.

Step 10 After three breaths, sit up and release your arms and legs. Stretch out before switching sides.

TARGET MUSCLES

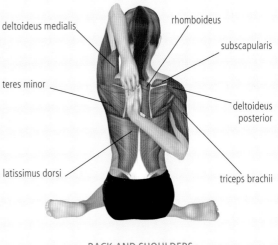

deltoideus medialis

rhomboideus

subscapularis

teres minor

deltoideus posterior

latissimus dorsi

triceps brachii

BACK AND SHOULDERS

CAUTIONS
- If you have knee pain, avoid this pose.
- If you have any shoulder issues, be carful of forcing your arms into position.

MODIFICATIONS

Sit on a blanket if your hips are tight or uncomfortable. Only do the legs or the arms. Use a strap for your arms.

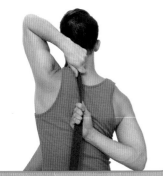

Pigeon Pose
Eka Pada Rajakapotasana

There are two stages to this hip opener. The first stage is more of a passive stretch. You fold forward focusing mainly on the stretch in the external hip rotators, glutes, and piriformis. The second stage requires strong engagement of the back muscles. As you begin to walk your hands back, start to gently bend your back. Remember to continue to lengthen your tailbone, and draw your belly button to your spine.

CAUTIONS
• If you have any knee problems, avoid this pose.

Step 1 From an extended Table pose, slide your right knee forward just behind your right wrist, and just outside the line of your right hip, with your shin on an angle under your torso. If your hips are open and flexible, place your shin parallel to the front of the mat.

Step 2 Putting weight into your hands and front shin, slowly stretch out through your back leg, resting your thigh on the mat, toes untucked. Peek back to check that your left leg points straight back and is internally rotated.

Step 3 Release your right buttock to the mat, making sure your front knee is comfortable and your hip points are even. Release your tailbone down and lengthen your lower back.

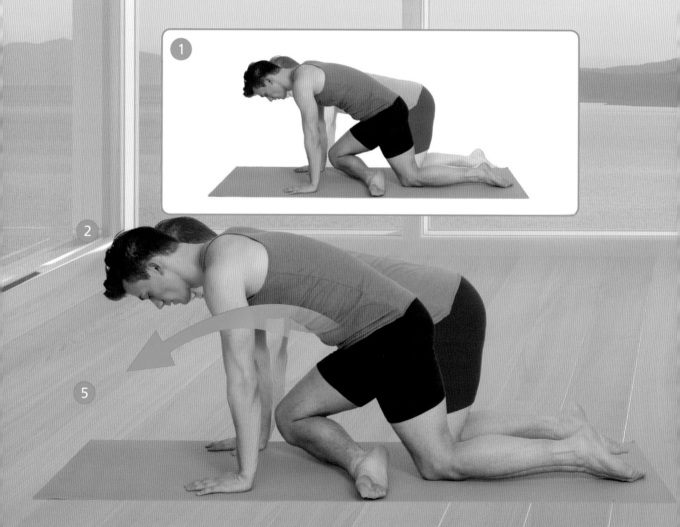

Step 4 Stretch up through your spine, draw your upper arms back, and draw your breastbone forward and up.

Step 5 Lower your torso down, leading with the chest. Rest your forehead on the mat, arms extended.

Step 6 After three breaths, lift your torso back up, walk your hands even further back, draw your belly button to your spine, and lengthen your tailbone. Lift up through your breastbone and draw your upper arms back.

Step 7 After three breaths, come back into the Table pose and stretch your right leg back, tuck your toes under, and press through your heel.

TARGET MUSCLES

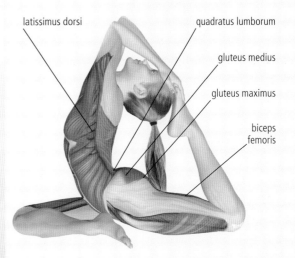

latissimus dorsi

quadratus lumborum

gluteus medius

gluteus maximus

biceps femoris

PIRIFORMIS AND GLUTES

MODIFICATION

Keep your front knee bent, and place that hip on a blanket for support.

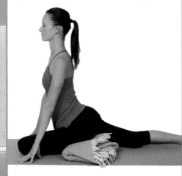

Half Lotus
Ardha Padmasana

The Lotus pose is the iconic meditation pose. For many, the Full Lotus pose is too challenging and precarious for the knees. Knee pain is usually related to inflexibilities in the hips. So just work on the Half Lotus. Remember to practice on both sides.

CAUTIONS
- If you have any knee issues, avoid this pose.

THINGS TO THINK ABOUT
- Foot inflexibility can also cause discomfort in this pose.

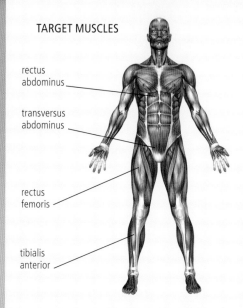

TARGET MUSCLES

rectus abdominus

transversus abdominus

rectus femoris

tibialis anterior

LEGS AND ABDOMINALS

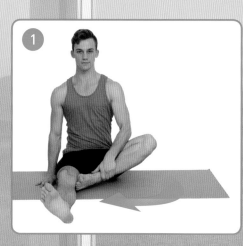

Step 1 Sit on a mat, and bend your left knee. Allow your left hip to open and lower your outer thigh to the floor.

Step 2 Bring your left foot to your left hip crease, with your sole angled upward.

Step 3 Bend your right knee and slide your right foot under your left thigh.

Step 4 Ground both sitz bones evenly as you extend upward through your spine and the crown of your head.

Step 5 Rest the backs of your hands on your knees.

Step 6 Carefully release, extending your legs straight, before doing the other side.

MODIFICATION

Sit on a blanket if you have tight hips.

Hero
Virasana

At first this pose looks easy—kids sit in this pose all the time. When adults begin to practice this pose, we feel major discomfort in our feet, shins, knees, and thighs. When practiced with alignment and props, there should be little sensation, if any at all. Props are very important here, so grab a couple and properly place them to regain flexibility in your legs.

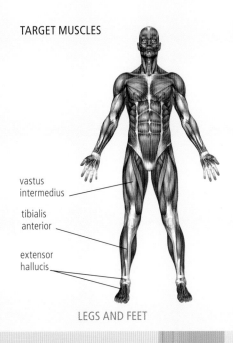

TARGET MUSCLES

vastus intermedius

tibialis anterior

extensor hallucis

LEGS AND FEET

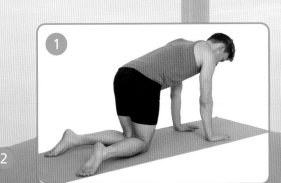

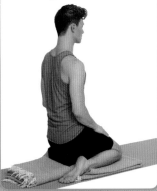

Step 1 Start in the Table pose. Bring your knees together, with your feet a little wider than your hips, and point your toes straight back.

Step 2 Use your hands to pull your calf muscles from your knee toward your ankle and out. Bring your hips back and sit on the floor between your feet.

Step 3 Pull aside your skin on the front of your knees.

Step 4 The soles of your feet face upward. Rotate your inner thighs.

Step 5 Place your hands on your thighs. Lift your spine and sit up tall.

Step 6 After a brief amount of time, come back into the Table pose and stretch out each leg by tucking your toes under and stretching your leg straight.

MODIFICATION

Sit on a folded blanket and pad your shins for tight feet.

CAUTIONS
- If you have any knee pain, avoid this pose.

THINGS TO THINK ABOUT
- Start with only one leg folded back, and then switch.

Hip Openers • 83

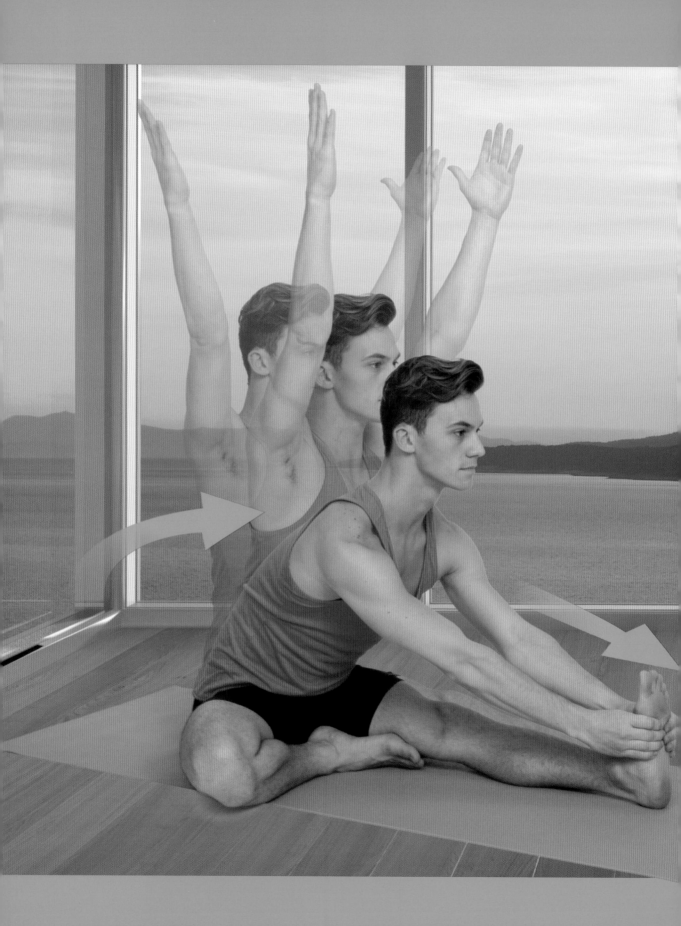

Forward Bends

Forward bends provide a powerful stretch to the entire back side of the body, from the heels to the back of the neck. This stretches, tones, and lengthens the entire spinal column, increasing flexibility in the spine and hips. Stretching muscles, ligaments, and nerves in the back of the legs can help alleviate certain cases of sciatica. These poses massage, oxygenate, and decongest the pelvis and abdominal organs. Forward bends relax the nervous system, thereby calming the mind and emotions.

Staff Pose
Dandasana

The Staff pose may look like just sitting, but when it is practiced with real intention, it is quite challenging. It may not be as exciting as some of the other poses, but it is important. Keep doing it.

Step 1 Sit on the floor with your legs stretched out in front, your feet a few inches apart.

Step 2 Flex your feet, stretch out through your inner heels, and draw the outer edges of your feet back toward you.

Step 3 Firm the muscles of your legs. Bring your fingertips just behind your buttocks while keeping your elbows soft.

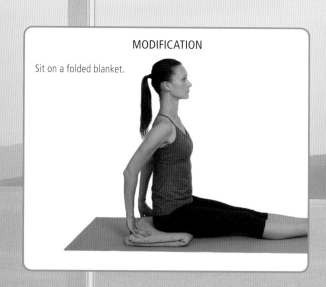

MODIFICATION

Sit on a folded blanket.

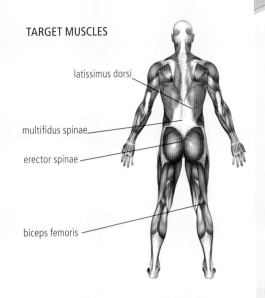

TARGET MUSCLES

latissimus dorsi

multifidus spinae

erector spinae

biceps femoris

BACK AND HAMSTRINGS

Step 4 Stretch down into your fingertips as you lift up through your spine. Move your upper arms back, shoulder blades together, and lift your breastbone, to expand your chest.

Step 5 After three breaths, relax out of the pose.

4

Half/Full Standing Forward Bend
Uttanasana /Ardha Uttanasana

Let gravity help you out in this basic forward bend. Feel a sense of release as you hang over, releasing and lengthening your spine, up through your neck and the muscles around the base of your head. The Half Standing Forward Bend develops strength and flexibility in the back of your legs, and in the back and core, to hold the torso away from gravity. This pose is sometimes incorporated into sun saluations.

Step 1 Stand on a mat, with your feet hip-width apart and parallel, and your hands on your hips.

Step 2 Inhale and lift your breastbone. Exhale and, hinged deep in your hip socket, fold forward, keeping your spine extended.

Step 3 Bring your fingertips to the floor (or blocks), shoulder-width apart.

CAUTIONS
• If you have a sensitive lower back, bend your knees and roll up to standing to exit the pose.

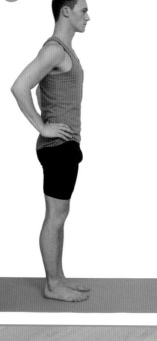

Step 4 Release your head and neck, while still grounding into all four corners of your feet, with your legs engaged.

Step 5 Place your hands on your shins, or your fingers on blocks below your shoulders. Engage your core. Inhale, press into your shins, and lift halfway up.

Step 6 Extend through your tailbone and out through the top of your head, and draw the shoulder blades toward each other on the back.

Step 7 Exhale and release as you stand upright.

Step 8 After three breaths, activate your legs, draw your belly button to your spine, and place your hands back on your hips. Draw your shoulders and elbows back to open your chest. With a flat back, inhale and come up.

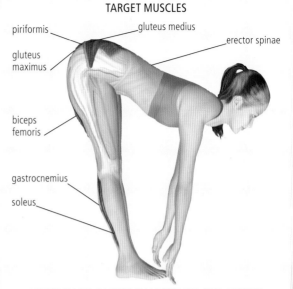

TARGET MUSCLES

piriformis

gluteus medius

erector spinae

gluteus maximus

biceps femoris

gastrocnemius

soleus

LOWER BACK, CALVES, HAMSTRINGS, AND GLUTES

4

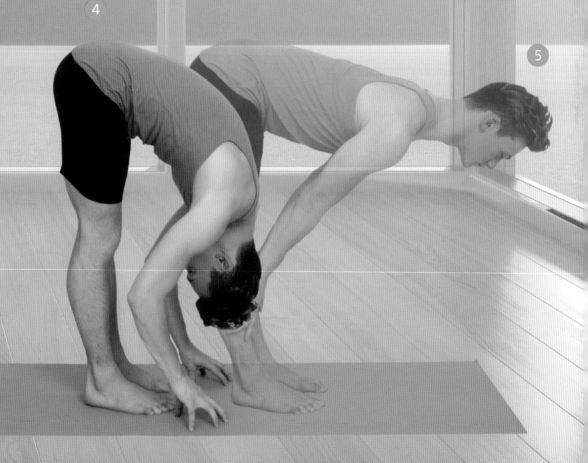

5

Head to Knees
Janu Sirsasana

Just because the name of this pose is "Head to Knees" doesn't mean your head has to be anywhere near your knees to get its benefits. This beginner forward bend stretches the back of one leg at a time, making the pose a little easier than a full forward bend with both legs in front. Keep the extended leg active, and focus on breathing in this pose.

Step 1 Sit on a mat.

Step 2 Bend your right knee. Release it out to the side and place the sole of your right foot on the inside of your left thigh.

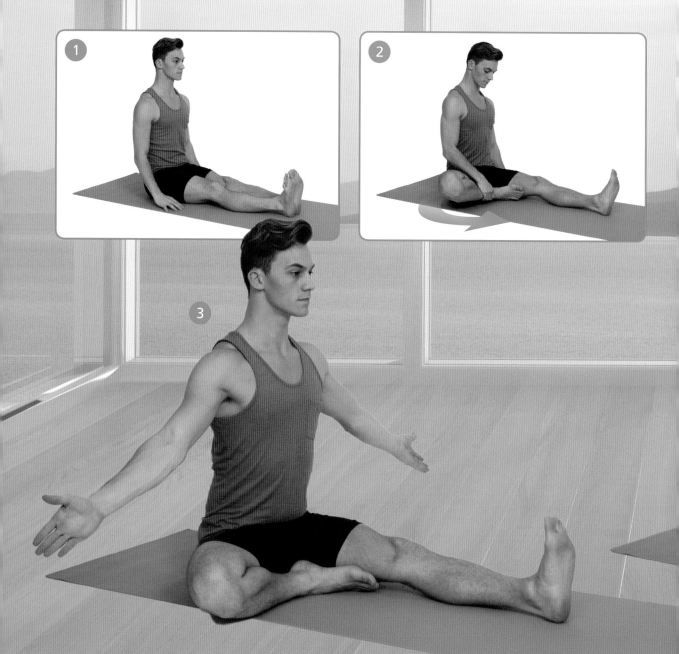

Step 3 Extend through your spine and activate the extended leg, with your foot flexed. Inhale and lift your arms overhead.

Step 4 On your exhale, hinge forward at the hips and take hold of your foot, ankle, or shin.

Step 5 Relax your neck and keep your head in line with your spine.

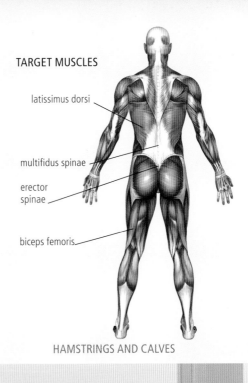

TARGET MUSCLES

latissimus dorsi

multifidus spinae

erector spinae

biceps femoris

HAMSTRINGS AND CALVES

Step 6 After three breaths, inhale and lengthen your spine. Reach your arms forward and up. Exhale and release your arms.

Step 7 Extend your legs back and sit upright.

CAUTIONS
- If you have any discomfort in your lower back, bend the knee of your extended leg, or use a strap.

THINGS TO THINK ABOUT
- The bent leg hip is also getting a stretch, along with the same inner groin.

MODIFICATION

If you have tight hamstrings, sit on a blanket and use a strap.

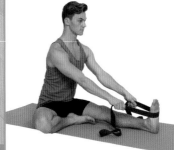

Seated Full Forward Bend
Paschimottanasana

Don't we always want to be able to touch our toes—isn't that the true measure of flexibility? Not really. If we compromise this pose just to touch our toes, we miss out on so much. Work slowly and precisely in this pose. Use any and all props to make this pose possible for you. Focus on hinging at the hips and keeping length in the spine rather than lurching forward and holding on.

Step 1 Sit on a mat. Activate your legs and flex the feet, drawing the outer edge of your foot toward you, with the big toe side facing away.

Step 2 Extend through your spine. Inhale and stretch up your arms.

Step 3 On an exhale, hinge forward at the hips, keeping your spine long. Take hold of your shins, ankles, or feet. Keep your neck in line with your spine.

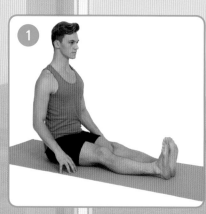

CAUTIONS
- If you have any discomfort in your lower back, bend your knees.

THINGS TO THINK ABOUT
- Your ego is going to take over here. Watch it. Remind yourself that you don't get a medal when you touch your toes. Be where you are.

Step 4 Relax your neck and head, keeping it in line with your spine.

Step 5 After three breaths, draw your belly button to your spine and reach your arms forward and up.

Step 6 Exhale. Release your arms to sit upright.

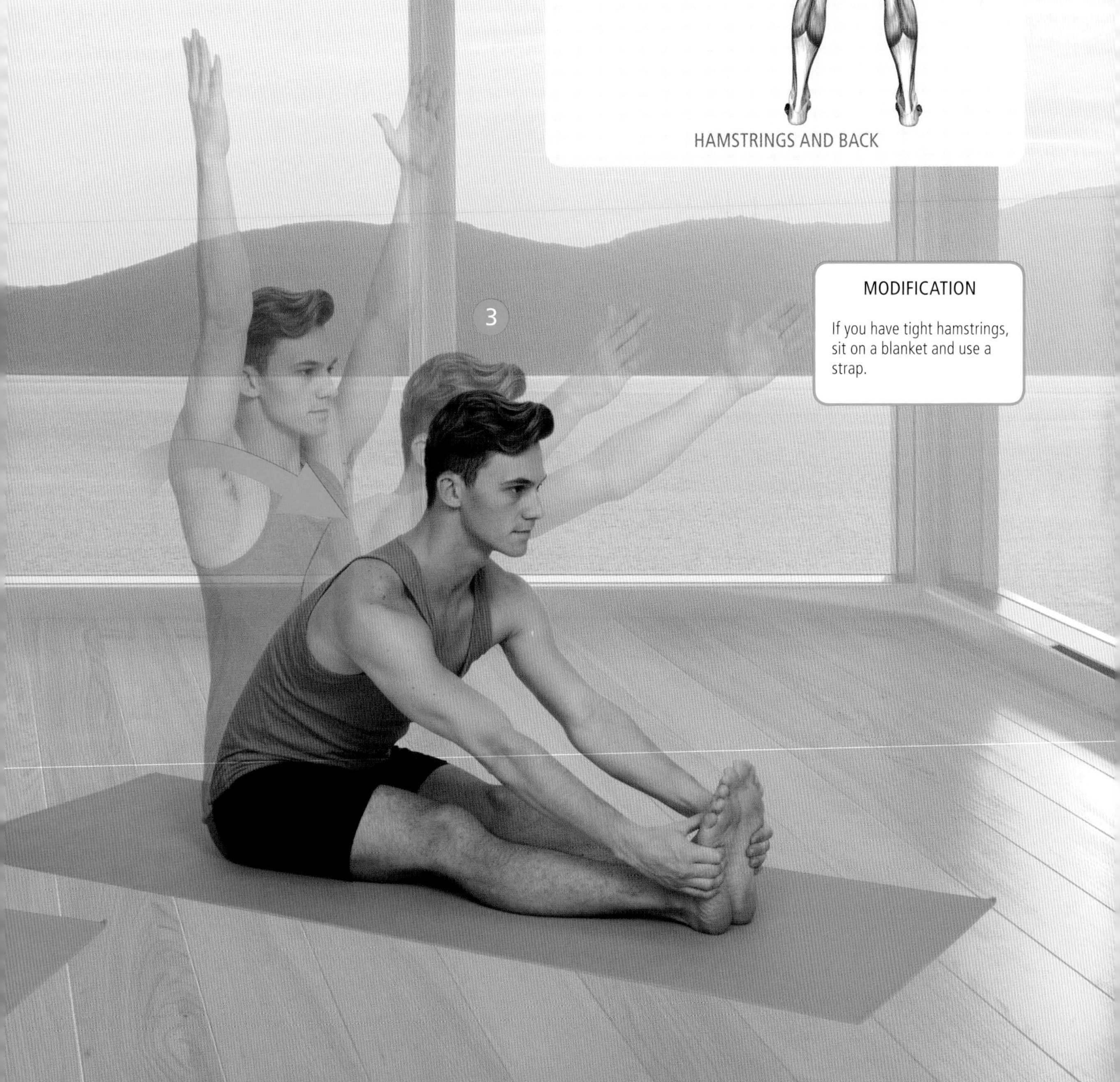

TARGET MUSCLES

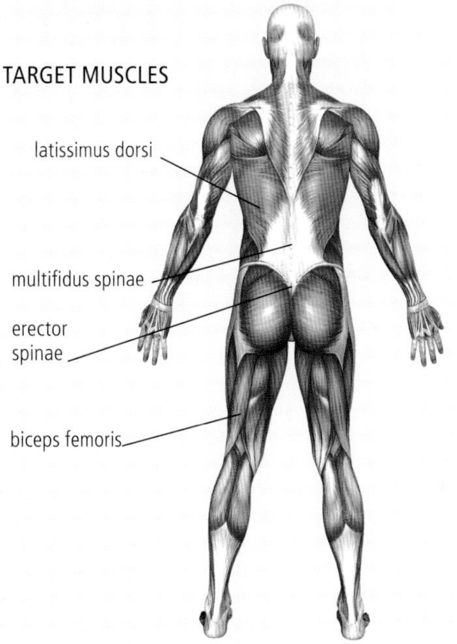

latissimus dorsi

multifidus spinae

erector spinae

biceps femoris

HAMSTRINGS AND BACK

3

MODIFICATION

If you have tight hamstrings, sit on a blanket and use a strap.

Wide-Angle Seated Forward Bend

Upavistha Konasana

This forward bend not only stretches out the back, but also adds the adductors (inner thigh muscles) into the mix, making this a more complicated forward bend. Beyond the physical aspects of this pose, it can be psychologically challenging. The mind gets active as we try to fold in a class, and thoughts about why we can't—or why our poses don't look like the poses of other students—cycle through the mind. At first you may not be able to bend forward much in this pose. Try to be very aware of the deep physical sensations and observe your thoughts as they arise.

Step 1 Sit with your legs open. Adjust your position until your sitting bones feel grounded. Pull the flesh of your buttocks back and aside. Stretch out through your heels, and keep your knees and second toe pointing straight up.

Step 2 Place your fingertips on the floor just behind your hips, with your elbows soft, and stretch through your spine and lift your breastbone.

1

CAUTIONS
- If you have any discomfort behind the knees, bring the legs closer together.

THINGS TO THINK ABOUT
- If pain continues behind the knees or the inner knees, slightly bend the knees and place a rolled towel under each one. Now engage the legs, pressing the back of the knees into the towel.

Step 3 Place your hands in front. Keep your spine long as you fold forward by gradually walking your hands forward.

Step 4 After three breaths, inhale and walk your hands back up to the seated position.

Step 5 Draw your legs back together and shake out.

TARGET MUSCLES

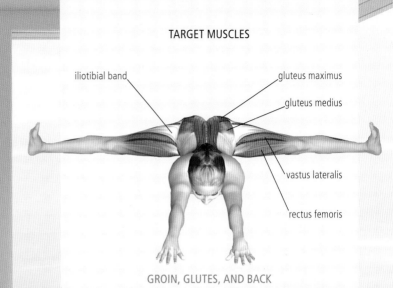

iliotibial band

gluteus maximus

gluteus medius

vastus lateralis

rectus femoris

GROIN, GLUTES, AND BACK

MODIFICATION

If you have tight hamstrings, sit on a blanket and don't fold.

3

Wide Leg Standing Forward Bend
Prasarita Padottanasana

This pose demands an energized effort from your lower body, to safely create the space to release and quiet the mind. Pretend you are standing on ice and you need to prevent your feet from sliding further out. Feel your legs hug your midline, while your torso and head soften toward the floor. Work to find a balance between these two energies.

Step 1 Stand sideways on your mat.

Step 2 Walk your feet wide enough so your heels would fall under your wrists if your arms were extended in a "T."

Step 3 Place your hands on your hips. Draw your shoulder blades together to open your chest.

CAUTIONS
- If you have any discomfort in the back of your knees, shift your weight toward your heels, narrow the stance, or bend your knees slightly.

MODIFICATION

If you have a tight back or hamstrings, place your hands on blocks.

Step 4 Inhale to lengthen. As you exhale, hinge from your hips and fold forward.

Step 5 Press into the outer edge of your feet while at the same time drawing your legs to your midline.

Step 6 If possible, release your head and neck and walk your fingertips through your legs.

Step 7 After three or four breaths, press into your feet, draw your belly button to your spine, place your hands back on your hips, and draw your elbows back, shoulder blades toward each other, and inhale as you lift back up.

Step 8 Release your hands and walk or hop your feet together.

TARGET MUSCLES

gluteus medius

obliquus externus

vastus lateralis

rectus femoris

teres major

soleus

flexor digitorum

extensor hallucis

vastus intermedius

vastus medialis

tibialis anterior

peroneus

flexor hallucis

adductor hallucis

OUTER LEGS, BACK, AND INNER LEGS

4

5

6

Upward-Facing Boat
Paripurna Navasana

This pose takes a considerable amount of core strength. Start where you need to: knees bent, fingers on the floor, or using a strap. Over time, you will build strength and stamina.

Step 1 Sit on the mat with your knees bent, the soles of your feet on the mat.

Step 2 Place your hands behind your hips, fingers pointing away from your feet. Lean back into your hands and lift your chest.

Step 3 Continue to lean back as you lift your feet off the floor and find a balance point on your buttocks.

Step 4 If possible, straighten your legs at a 45-degree angle to the floor.

Step 5 Point through your toes and reach your arms forward, parallel to the floor.

Step 6 Keep your belly button drawn into your spine, and relax your jaw and shoulders.

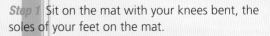

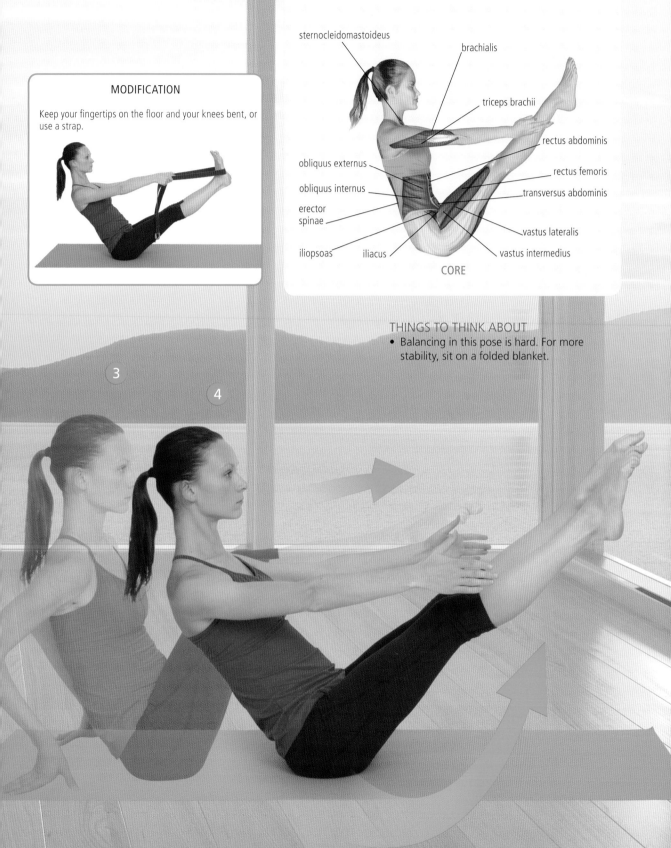

MODIFICATION

Keep your fingertips on the floor and your knees bent, or use a strap.

TARGET MUSCLES

sternocleidomastoideus

brachialis

triceps brachii

rectus abdominis

obliquus externus

rectus femoris

obliquus internus

transversus abdominis

erector spinae

vastus lateralis

iliopsoas

iliacus

vastus intermedius

CORE

THINGS TO THINK ABOUT
• Balancing in this pose is hard. For more stability, sit on a folded blanket.

3

4

Standing Split
Urdhva Prasarita Eka Padasana

It is tempting to put all your focus into lifting your raised leg higher. Try not to get wrapped up in that, and put equal focus on your standing leg. Wherever your raised leg is, keep your leg and foot active. You can add more balance play to this pose by grasping your standing ankle with one hand.

Step 1 Stand in the Mountain pose. Shift your weight into your left foot, being conscious to evenly distribute the weight on all four corners of your foot and activate your legs.

Step 2 With a flat back, hinge forward at your hips and lift your right leg behind you.

Step 3 Keep your shoulders and hips square as you reach your fingertips toward the floor (or blocks).

Step 4 The tendency is to open the right hip to the ceiling. Try to have both hip points facing the mat.

Step 5 If possible, play with balance by grasping one or both of your hands around your left ankle.

Step 6 Draw your belly button to your spine, and come back to a standing position.

THINGS TO THINK ABOUT
- As you press down into your standing leg and foot, lift your upper leg away from the floor, and extend it toward the sky.

MODIFICATION

Place your hands on blocks.

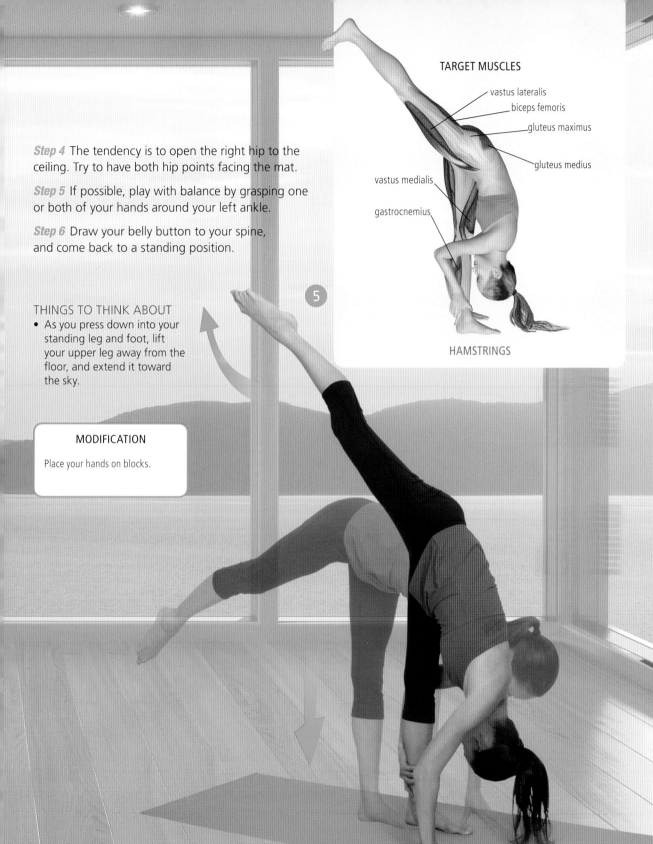

TARGET MUSCLES

vastus lateralis

biceps femoris

gluteus maximus

gluteus medius

vastus medialis

gastrocnemius

HAMSTRINGS

5

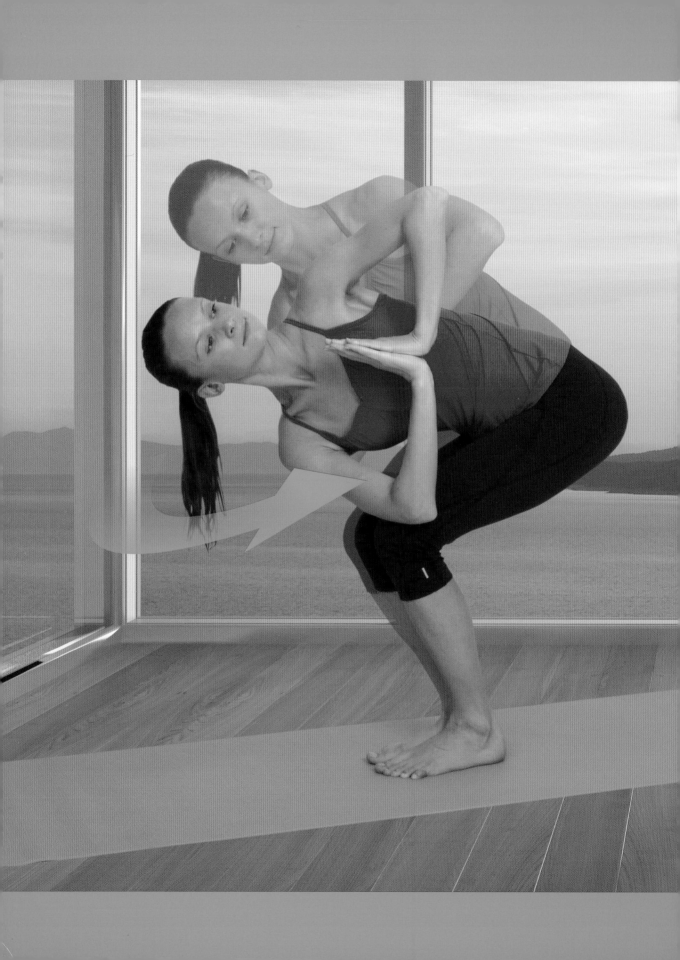

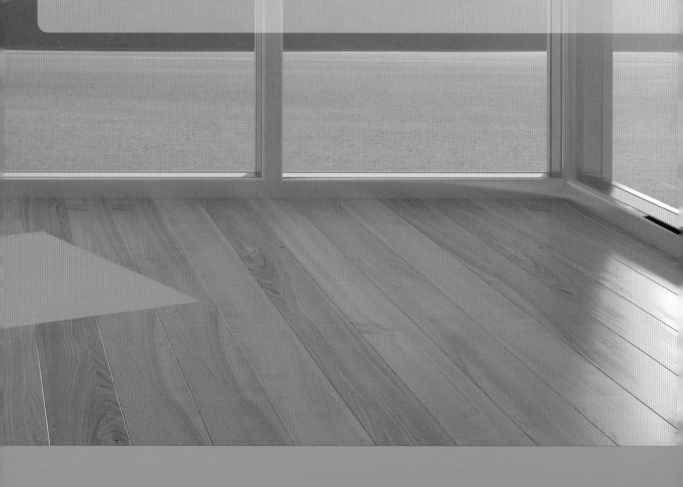

Twisted Poses

Twists rotate, extend, and align the spine, helping to inhibit the spinal
fusing and immobility that frequently happens as we age. Twists hydrate
spinal disks and keep them healthy. They also enhance circulation of blood
and oxygen to the entire musculoskeletal system along the spine. Twists
are useful in helping to correct deviation or scoliosis in the spinal column.
They can relieve stiffness, back strain, and certain forms of sciatica.
Twists have a neutralizing effect on the nervous system, helping to
rejuvenate the entire body/mind and creating a sense of well-being.

Simple Seated Twist
Bharadvajasana

This is an open twist, allowing for more of the spine to twist with ease. While there is a natural tendency to bend back in this pose, be mindful of popping your lower ribs. Keep lengthening through the crown of your head as your lower body grounds you.

Step 1 Sit on a mat. Tuck your feet and legs off to the right. Allow your knees to splay, with your toes pointing back and your top ankle sitting in the arch of your bottom foot.

Step 2 Drop your right sitz bone, trying to level the left and right—use a folded blanket placed under your left sitz bone to help if you can't sit evenly.

Step 3 Sit tall and place your right hand on your left knee, and your left hand behind your fingers, pointing away.

Step 4 Keep your spine neutral as you twist to the left, looking over your left shoulder. Avoid swaying your back.

Step 5 After three breaths, exhale and release the twist, and face forward.

THINGS TO THINK ABOUT
- As you inhale, lift your spine; as you exhale, twist a little bit deeper. Continue, making sure you are always able to breathe easily.

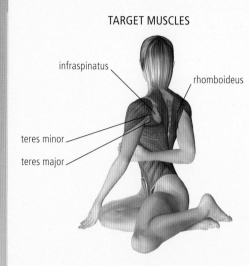

TARGET MUSCLES

infraspinatus

rhomboideus

teres minor

teres major

BACK

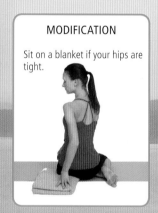

MODIFICATION

Sit on a blanket if your hips are tight.

Supine Twist
Jathara Parivartanasana

The Supine Twist is a gentle twist to neutralize the spine. There are many variations that can make this pose more challenging, but before moving deeper, stop and listen to the sensations of your body to determine if moving deeper is safe and appropriate.

Step 1 Lie on your back with your arms extended into a T position. Bend your knees toward your chest and flex your feet.

Step 2 Inhale, and as you exhale, drop your knees across your body to the left side, rolling onto your left hip.

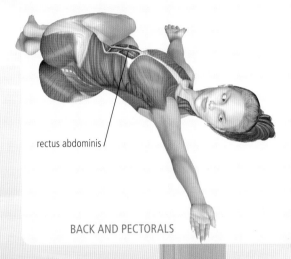

TARGET MUSCLES

rectus abdominis

BACK AND PECTORALS

Step 3 Try to keep your right shoulder blade, arm, and upper back grounded, and stretch through your fingertips.

Step 4 After three to four breaths, inhale and use your abdominals to bring your torso and knees back to the center, before twisting to the other side.

THINGS TO THINK ABOUT
- This is a simple, easy twist that most everyone can do. Even though it may feel simple, you still benefit by doing this pose. Add it toward the end to all your sequences to help wind down before deep relaxation.

Marichi's Pose
Marichyasana III

Seated twisting poses stretch and strengthen the back and core muscles, while giving the internal organs a massage. The bent knee acts as a fulcrum to deepen the twist. Make sure your weight is evenly distributed in both sitz bones throughout this pose. Twists are another great place to focus on breathing: inhale to lengthen and exhale to twist.

Step 1 Sit on a mat.

Step 2 Bend your left knee, bringing your heel toward your buttock. Activate your right leg and stretch through your heel.

Step 3 Place your hands at either side. Using gentle pressure into your fingertips, inhale and elongate your spine. Wrap your right hand around your left outer knee.

Step 4 Place your right hand a few inches behind your tailbone, with your fingertips on the floor pointing outward, elbow slightly bent. Inhale, and then as you exhale, twist toward the bent knee.

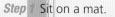

Step 5 Stretch up through your spine, lift your breastbone, and draw your left shoulder back.

Step 6 Gaze toward your left shoulder.

Step 7 Inhale, lift up, and twist to the left as you exhale. Continue to engage the upper back muscles. Lift and expand your chest.

Step 8 Be sure to twist from your belly button and bottom ribs to protect your lower back.

Step 9 Gently unwind, and prepare to repeat on the other side.

THINGS TO THINK ABOUT
- When holding your knee, keep from "gripping" your knee. Hold with a sense of purpose and intention.

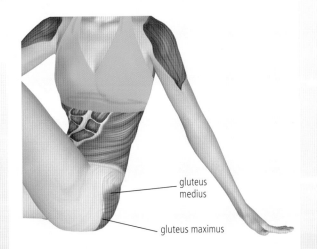

TARGET MUSCLES

gluteus medius

gluteus maximus

OUTER HIP, PIRIFORMIS, AND GLUTES

4

Half Spinal Twist
Ardha Matsyendrasana

This deep twist helps to balance the spine and its muscles, tendons, and ligaments. The crossed leg in this twist provides deeper massage to your internal organs. As you move from one side to the other, the squeeze and release brings more blood flow to those organs and squeezes out the toxins.

CAUTIONS
• If you have any discomfort in the lower back or sacrum, focus the twist higher up, modify, or avoid this pose.

Step 1 Sit on the floor with your legs stretched out in front of you in the Staff pose.

Step 2 Bend your left knee and place the sole of your foot outside of your right knee or thigh. Activate your right leg and stretch through your heel.

Step 3 Keep both sitting bones grounded, bend your right leg, with the outer edge of your thigh resting on the floor, your heel at the outer edge of your left hip.

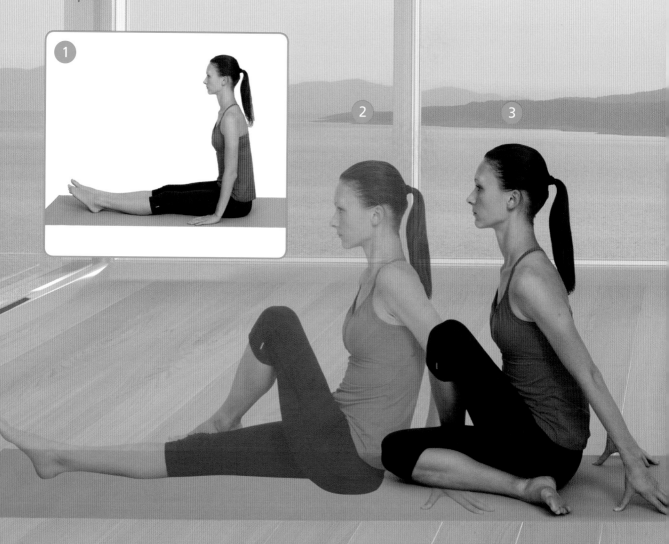

Step 4 Wrap your right arm around your left knee, and place your left hand a few inches behind your tailbone, with your fingertips on the floor pointing outward, elbow slightly bent. Stretch up through your spine, lift your breastbone, and draw your left shoulder back.

Step 5 Inhale and lift up. As you exhale, twist to the left. Continue to engage your upper back muscles. Lift and expand your chest.

Step 6 After three or four breaths, exhale and release the twist and face forward. Return to the Staff pose before setting up to twist to the other side.

MODIFICATION

If both sitting bones don't sit on the floor, straighten your bottom leg, and/or sit on a blanket.

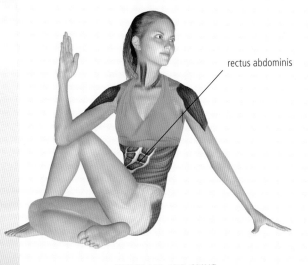

TARGET MUSCLES

rectus abdominis

OUTER HIP AND SPINE

4

5

Twisting Chair
Parivrtta Utkatasana

This standing twist is more challenging because you must work to keep the alignment as your legs tire. Focus on keeping your hips facing forward and your knees in line as you perform the twist.

Step 1 Start in the Chair pose. Bring your hands to prayer. Inhale here, and as you exhale, twist to the left.

Step 2 Keep lengthening your spine from your tailbone to the crown of your head. Hook your right elbow against your outer left thigh.

Step 3 Check that your knees are still in line—the tendency is for the right knee to move forward. Level your knees and hips.

Step 4 Draw your shoulder blades together in your back to open your chest.

Step 5 Inhale. As you exhale, release the twist and return to the Chair pose.

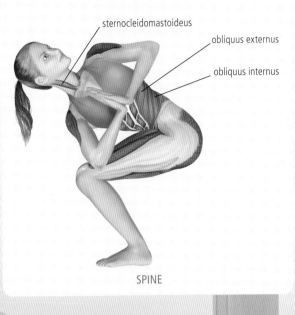

TARGET MUSCLES

sternocleidomastoideus

obliquus externus

obliquus internus

SPINE

THINGS TO THINK ABOUT
- To deepen the twist and keep your balance, press your outer thigh into your upper arm, and press your upper arm into your outer thigh.

2

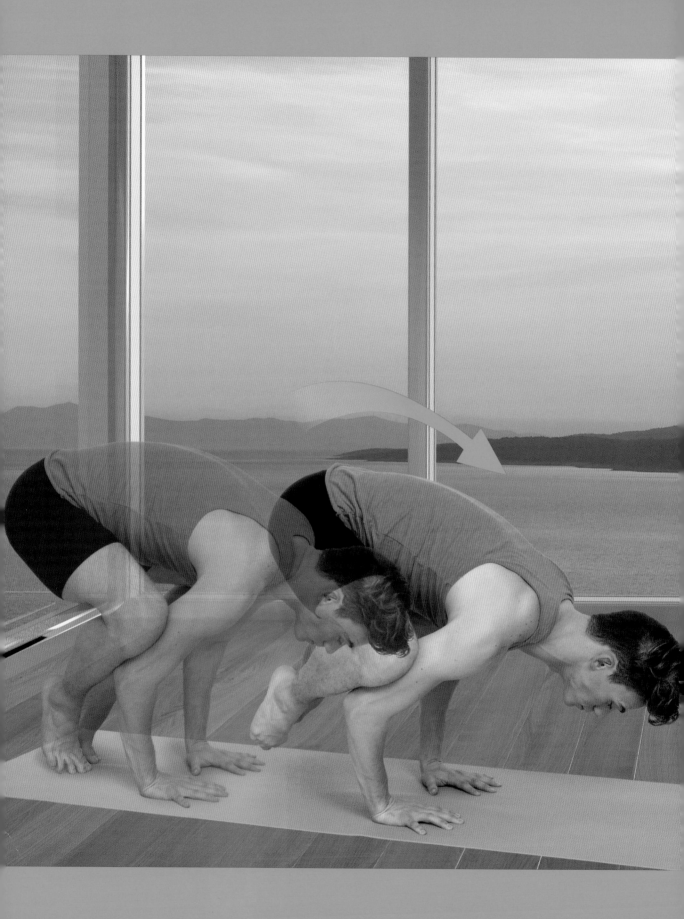

Arm Balances and Inversions

Arm balances and inversions require a combination of strength and flexibility. You need abdominal strength to support and stabilize the center of your body—these poses challenge us, while testing our focus and perseverance. With gravity's pull on us throughout our lives, it's nice to take a moment to flip it all over. Inversions improve the flow of blood and energy to the brain, stimulate mental functions, improve memory and concentration, and can relieve some headaches. They also nourish the facial skin, scalp, and hair roots. Because of the reverse effect of gravity, internal organs get lifted out of their space, and edema and varicose veins get relief, as fluids flow without strain.

Upward Table/Plank
Purvottanasana

This pose is a great counter pose to all the forward bends. It opens up the front body by stretching the shoulders, chest, and abdomen. It also increases strength in the shoulders, arms, legs, glutes, and wrists. It is a challenging but invigorating pose.

Step 1 Begin in the Staff pose (sitting upright, legs stretched out in front of you). Place your hands several inches behind your hips, with your fingers pointing toward your toes. Bend your knees, placing the soles of your feet flat on the mat.

Step 2 Lean back into your hands. Bend your elbows and draw your shoulder blades together, opening your chest. Press into your feet and straighten your arms, lifting your hips into the Reverse Table pose.

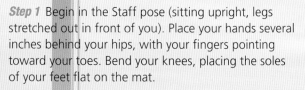

Step 3 Check the alignment of your shoulders over your wrists, and your knees over your ankles. Keeping your hips lifted, straighten each leg, press your heels into the floor, and lift your hips up without overly firming your buttocks.

Step 4 If it is comfotable for your neck, you can drop your head back, opening your throat.

Step 5 Take three breaths and feel a stretch from the tops of your feet, all along your front body. Allow your back to support the opening.

Step 6 To release, bring your head back to neutral and slowly lower back to the Staff pose.

TARGET MUSCLES

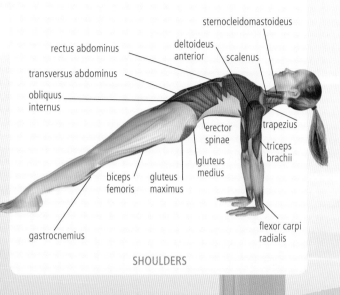

rectus abdominus
transversus abdominus
obliquus internus
sternocleidomastoideus
deltoideus anterior
scalenus
erector spinae
trapezius
triceps brachii
gluteus medius
biceps femoris
gluteus maximus
gastrocnemius
flexor carpi radialis

SHOULDERS

CAUTIONS
- If you have wrist or shoulder pain, modify or avoid this pose.

THINGS TO THINK ABOUT
- Once you are in the pose, reengage your feet and press up through your hips to get height.

③

MODIFICATIONS

If your wrists bother you, turn your hands out. Bend your knees for extra support.

Plank

The Plank is a foundational pose. It builds strength all over your body. Your strengths and weaknesses show up quickly in this pose. Do you arch your lower back or round your upper back? Focus on getting the alignment right even if you can only hold it for a few breaths at first.

Step 1 Start in a long Table pose (hands one hand's length ahead of shoulders), with your toes tucked.

Step 2 With your fingers spread and arms engaged, draw your belly button to your spine. Press back through your heels as you lift your knees away from the mat.

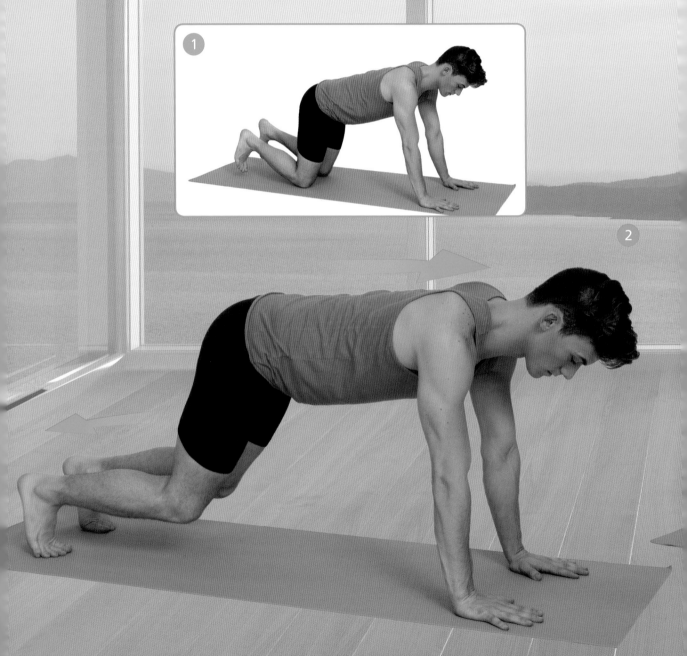

Step 3 Keep your body in one long line, heels pressing back, breastbone moving forward, opening your chest. Think of a mild upper back bend.

Step 4 Take three breaths. Either press your hips up and back into the Downward Dog or lower your knees to the mat and rest in the Table pose.

CAUTIONS
- If you experience wrist pain, check that your hands are pointing forward.
- If your wrists are pointing forward and you have wrist pain, either shift your weight back onto your toes or avoid this exercise.

MODIFICATION
Put your knees on the floor in a long Table pose.

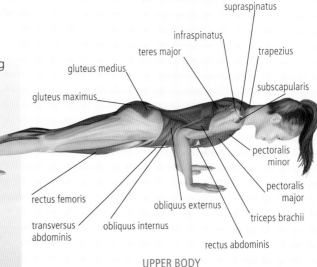

TARGET MUSCLES

suprastinatus

infraspinatus

teres major

trapezius

gluteus medius

subscapularis

gluteus maximus

pectoralis minor

pectoralis major

rectus femoris

obliquus externus

triceps brachii

transversus abdominis

obliquus internus

rectus abdominis

UPPER BODY

3

Side Plank
Vasisthasana

The Side Plank strengthens the shoulders, arms, wrists, and obliques. The action of pressing down with your hands and feet counters the lift of the hips and torso. You can only go up by pressing down first.

CAUTIONS
- If there is wrist pain, check that your fingers are pointing forward. Draw muscular energy up from your wrist to the armpit.

THINGS TO THINK ABOUT
- Your hips want to dip toward the floor, so keep your legs engaged and lift your shins away from the floor, too.

Step 1 Begin in the Plank pose.

Step 2 Shift your weight into your left hand as you roll onto the outside of your left foot. Externally rotate your left upper arm as you draw your left shoulder blade onto your back.

TARGET MUSCLES

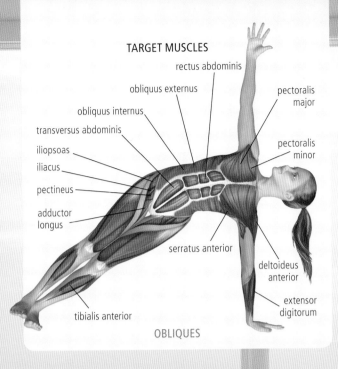

rectus abdominis

obliquus externus

obliquus internus

transversus abdominis

iliopsoas

iliacus

pectineus

adductor
longus

serratus anterior

tibialis anterior

pectoralis
major

pectoralis
minor

deltoideus
anterior

extensor
digitorum

OBLIQUES

MODIFICATIONS

Place your top leg foot on the floor in front of you for support.
Rest on your forearm instead
of your wrist on the floor.

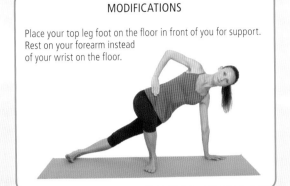

Step 3 Stack your feet and hips, press into your feet,
activate and squeeze your legs together to lift your hips.
Place your right hand on the hip. Once you have your
balance, reach your right hand up to the ceiling and gaze
up at your right fingertips.

Step 4 With control, return to the Plank pose.

3

Four-Limbed Staff Pose
Chaturanga Dandasana

This pose is most commonly used as a transitional pose in a sun salutation. It takes a lot of upper-body and core strength to perform correctly. As you begin to work this pose, start by lowering only so far as you can keep your shoulders from dipping forward.

CAUTION
• If you have any shoulder pain, please avoid this pose.

THINGS TO THINK ABOUT
• Keep your tailbone moving toward your heels and your breastbone moving forward. Try not to tip your shoulders toward the floor.

MODIFICATION
Place your knees on the floor.

FLOW

Flow from the Upward Dog to the Downward Dog.

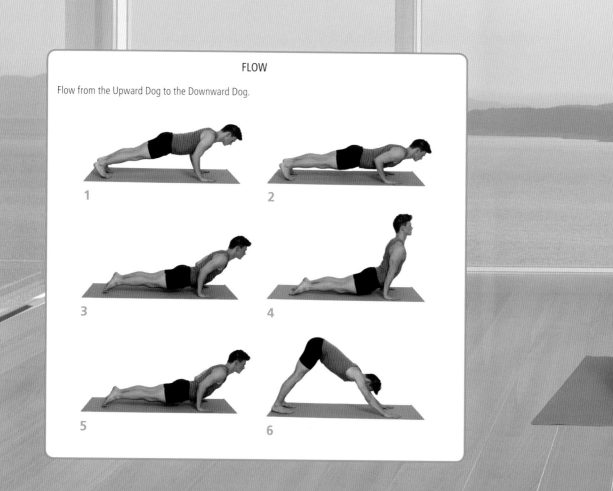

1

2

3

4

5

6

Step 1 From the Plank, draw your shoulder blades toward each other, with your breastbone moving forward. Draw your tailbone down and your pubic bone toward your navel so your lower back does not sag. Press out through your heels.

Step 2 Slowly lower your torso toward the mat, keeping your elbows squeezed close to your body. Hold when your upper arms are parallel to the floor. Draw your breastbone forward and press out though your heels. Keep your hips lifted in line with your shoulders and feet.

Step 3 Release to your stomach and rest.

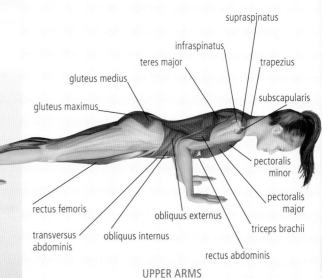

TARGET MUSCLES

supraspinatus

infraspinatus

teres major

gluteus medius

gluteus maximus

trapezius

subscapularis

pectoralis minor

pectoralis major

rectus femoris

obliquus externus

triceps brachii

transversus abdominis

obliquus internus

rectus abdominis

UPPER ARMS

Crow
Bakasana

The Crow is a challenging but accessible introductory arm balance. Try to have a playful sense of humor as you work this pose. Teeter forward and back to eventually find your balance point. Making yourself as compact as possible is key to lifting yourself up off the floor.

Step 1 Begin in a squat with your feet together and your inner big toes and heels touching. Lean forward, placing your hands, fingers spread, on the floor a couple inches in front of you, shoulder-width apart.

Step 2 Bend your elbows, creating a shelf with your upper arms. Draw your knees up into your armpits and squeeze your knees to your midline.

THINGS TO THINK ABOUT
- When engaging your core, legs, and arms, think about lifting yourself from deep inside.
- If you have shoulder and wrist pain, modify or avoid this pose.

Step 3 Draw in your belly button to your spine, make yourself compact, and perch on your tiptoes.

Step 4 Lean forward, bringing more weight into your hands and your shins to your upper arms.

Step 5 Continue to engage your core, squeezing your legs and and lifting your toes off the ground one foot at a time, finding your balance point. Then bring your big toes and inner heels together.

Step 6 Slowly release your feet back to the mat or jump back to the Four-Limbed Staff pose.

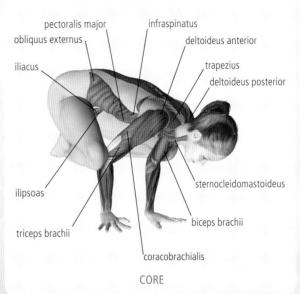

TARGET MUSCLES

pectoralis major
obliquus externus
iliacus
infraspinatus
deltoideus anterior
trapezius
deltoideus posterior
sternocleidomastoideus
ilipsoas
biceps brachii
triceps brachii
coracobrachialis

CORE

MODIFICATION

Perch your feet on blocks.

3

5

Side Crow
Parsva Bakasana

Once you are able to balance in the Crow pose, why not throw in a twist? This is a real yoga party trick! The key is not being afraid to fall. Go for it—you're not that far from the ground if you fall. You can even put a blanket out as a landing pad. This one is sure to bring a smile to your face once you find your perch.

Step 1 Squat down on your tiptoes, keeping your knees together. Twist to the left, hooking your right upper arm on the outside of your left outer thigh.

Step 2 Place your hands on the mat, shoulder-width apart, with your left hand in line with your outer thigh.

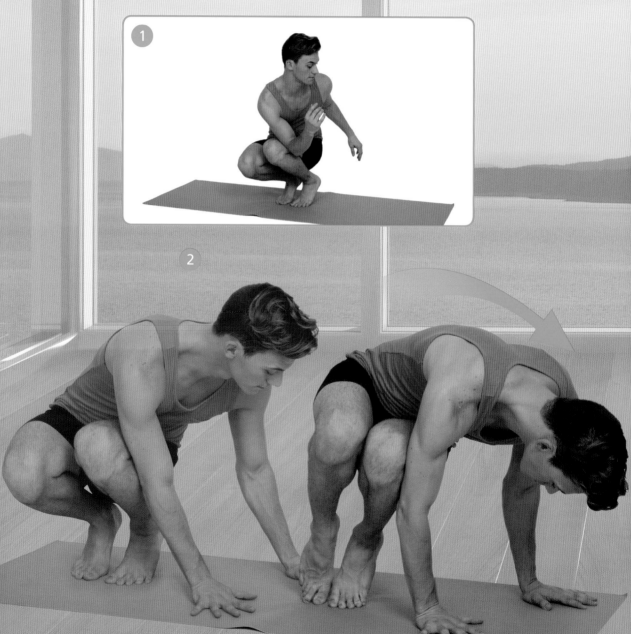

Step 3 Rest your outer right thigh on your left upper arm. Lean to the right and keep your arms firmly engaged as you bend your elbows and transfer your weight into your hands.

Step 4 Keep your feet together and draw your heels toward your buttocks.

Step 5 Slowly lower your feet to the floor, and very carefully unwind.

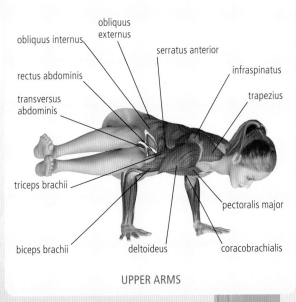

TARGET MUSCLES

obliquus internus

obliquus externus

serratus anterior

rectus abdominis

infraspinatus

transversus abdominis

trapezius

triceps brachii

pectoralis major

biceps brachii

deltoideus

coracobrachialis

UPPER ARMS

CAUTIONS
• If you have shoulder or wrist pain, avoid this pose.

THINGS TO THINK ABOUT
• To lift your legs and feet, squeeze them together and draw your energy up into your belly button.

Legs-up-the-Wall
Viparit Karani

This is the most basic inversion pose there is. It's not the most graceful pose to get into, but the key is getting your buttocks as close to the wall as possible from the start. Feel free to put a blanket under your hips or your head if it makes the pose more comfortable for you. You can also experiment with a belt around your thighs or an eye pillow over your eyes. Stay in the pose as long as is comfortable.

Step 1 Sit as close to the wall as you can, with your knees tucked into your chest.

Step 2 Turn sideways and lie down, simultaneously swinging your legs up the wall.

Step 3 Scoot your buttocks to the wall and extend your legs, feet flexed, heels resting on the wall.

Step 4 Relax your hands out to the side, palms up.

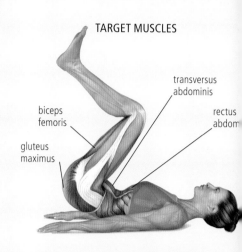

TARGET MUSCLES

transversus abdominis

biceps femoris

rectus abdom

gluteus maximus

ABDOMINALS, GLUTES, AND HAMSTRINGS

THINGS TO THINK ABOUT
- Allow gravity to drop your leg bones into your pelvis, and release your spine and head into the floor.
- Place a blanket under your hips if your hamstrings are tight. Place a folded blanket under your head.

MODIFICATION

If your hamstrings are tight, increase the height of the blanket, or move a couple of inches away from the wall.

"L" at the Wall

The "L" at the Wall is a great pose for all ages. It is considered a prep for the handstand but is also a great pose in and of itself. At first, if you are lined up correctly, you may feel like you are too close to the wall. That is natural. You can start with your feet higher up the wall to make it easier. As you build strength and confidence, inch your feet down the wall so your body forms a 90-degree angle. Relax your head and neck but keep your core engaged so your lower back doesn't sway.

Step 1 Kneel in the Table pose with your feet at the wall. Externally rotate and engage your upper arms. Draw your belly button to your spine, and press your hips up to a short Downward Dog pose, with your heels up the wall. Step one foot high up the wall, and then the other.

Step 2 Gradually walk your feet down so your heels are in line with your buttocks and your body forms an "L."

Step 3 Keep externally rotating your upper arms and pressing your belly button to your spine so that your back does not sway.

Step 4 Carefully step one foot down and then the other and rest in the Child's pose.

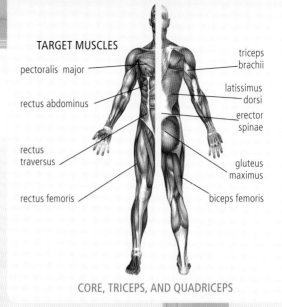

TARGET MUSCLES

- triceps brachii
- pectoralis major
- latissimus dorsi
- rectus abdominus
- erector spinae
- rectus traversus
- gluteus maximus
- rectus femoris
- biceps femoris

CORE, TRICEPS, AND QUADRICEPS

CAUTIONS
- If you have any wrist pain, avoid this pose.

THINGS TO THINK ABOUT
- Keep your tailbone moving up toward the ceiling, and drop your head.

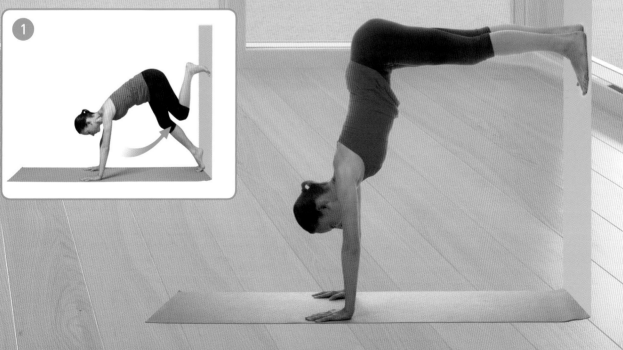

Supported Shoulder Stand
Salamba Sarvangasana

The setup for this pose may seem a bit prop-heavy, but don't skimp! The props are necessary to keep the neck in a safe alignment. The Shoulder Stand is often considered the "mother of all poses" because of its potential benefits, but it is challenging to get in and out of safely. Beginners should work up to this pose, and only perform it when they can do so without feeling strain on the neck.

Step 1 Prepare the setup as shown. Be sure when you lie down that your neck is on the smooth-edge fold of the blankets.

Step 2 Lie centered on your blankets, knees bent, buttocks on a block, feet on the floor, and your arms by your sides. Your shoulders should be roughly 2 inches from the edge of the blankets.

Step 3 With momentum, swing your knees toward your head, forming a tight ball, and catch your lower back with your hands.

Step 4 Rock from side to side, working your shoulders and elbows closer together under your body. Walk your hands toward your shoulder blades to support and lift your spine. Hook your hands around your outer waist.

Step 5 Keeping your knees bent, point your knees to the ceiling. Then stretch your legs up. Move your chin slightly away from your chest and soften your jaw. Stretch your tailbone toward your heels. Keep your gaze soft and around your knees. Do not turn your head to either side. Hold for approximately one minute.

CAUTIONS
• Do not practice this if you have any head, neck, or back issues.
• When in the pose, do not move your head.

THINGS TO THINK ABOUT
• Keep your chin moving away from your chest, and your gaze directly up by your knees.
• Props are absolutely necessary in this pose to keep your neck safe!

Step 6 To exit, bend your knees toward your face.

Step 7 Look back. Use your abdominal strength and the support of your hands to roll out of the pose. Keep your knees bent and place your feet on the floor.

Step 8 Slide back in the direction of your head, until your buttocks are sitting on the edge of the blankets where your shoulders were and your back is on the floor. Rest your heels on the edge of the blankets wider than your hips. Lean your knees together, then take your arms out to your sides, palms up.

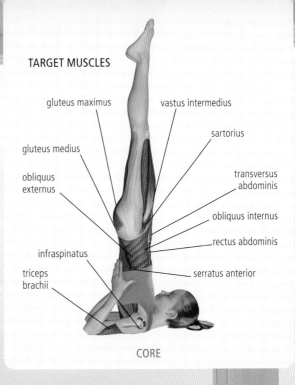

TARGET MUSCLES

gluteus maximus
vastus intermedius
sartorius
gluteus medius
transversus abdominis
obliquus externus
obliquus internus
rectus abdominis
infraspinatus
serratus anterior
triceps brachii

CORE

FLOW

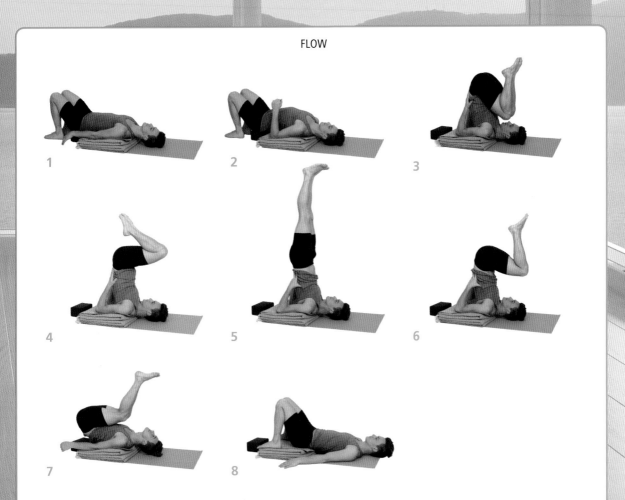

1
2
3
4
5
6
7
8

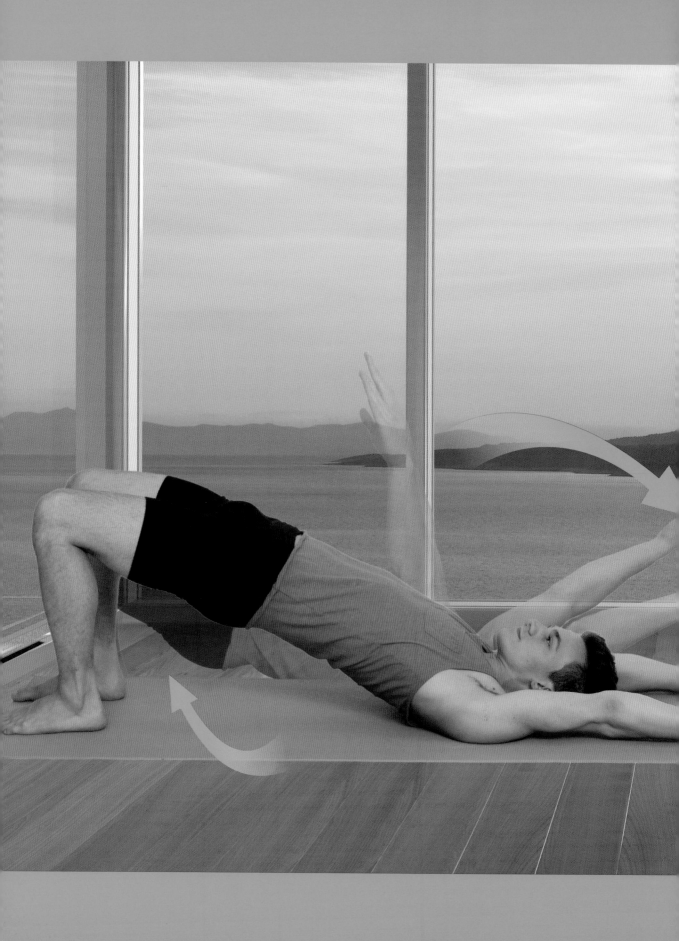

Movement and Breath

These poses may be simple, but the goal is to coordinate your breathing with the movement. Try to make the length of your inhale/exhale match the length of the movement. If you find you are still moving and you are already at the top of the breath, move slower. Become conscious of the comfortable length of your inhale and exhale, and fit your movements into that amount of time. Allow your breathing to direct your action.

Moving Bridge

Step 1 Lie on your back. Bend your knees and place your feet hip-width apart and parallel. Place your hands down by your sides, palms facing down.

Step 2 On your next inhale, lift your hips and arms up over your head. Try to gauge how long the inhale is going to be, and time your movements accordingly.

Step 3 At the top of the inhale, your hips should be up, and your arms should be up over your head by the floor, plams facing upward.

Step 4 Begin your exhale and start moving your arms back down, and your hips back to the floor. Both movements should end around the same time.

Step 5 Complete up to five rounds of this, ending with your hips down, and your hands on the floor by your hips. Return your breathing back to your natural rhythm, and soak in the sense of relaxation that comes over your body and mind.

THINGS TO THINK ABOUT
- As you get more comfortable and familiar coordinating your breath and actions, both will become more automatic.
- Enjoy the gentle wave as it moves up through your breath and body.

FLOW

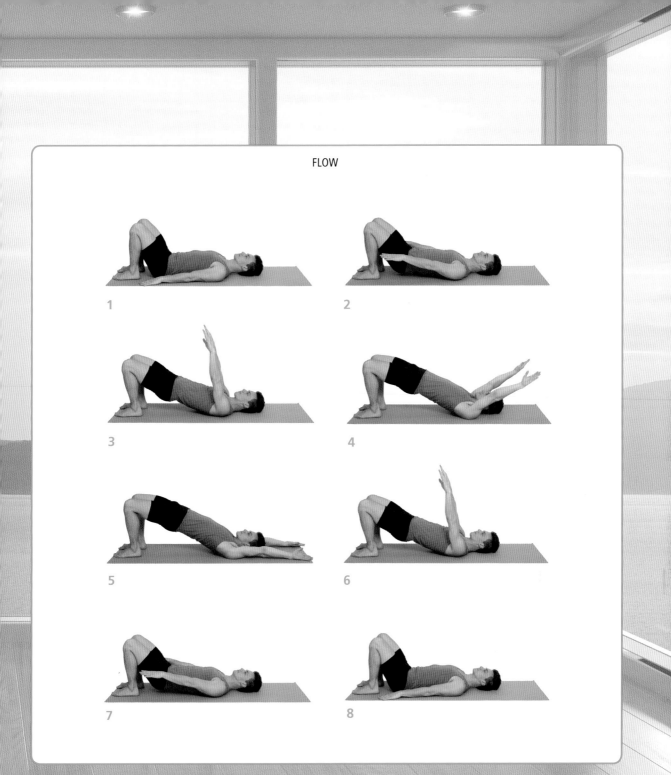

Flowing Downward Dog

Step 1 Start in the Downward Dog. Make sure you have even weight in both arms and legs. Your hands should be spread and steady, and your lower abdominals should be drawn in.

Step 2 On your inhale, lift your right leg up behind you into the Downward Dog split. Your leg should be extended, your foot should be flexed, and your toes pointing down.

Step 3 On your exhale, shifting into a Plank, bend your right knee and draw your knee toward your nose. Keep your knee and leg lifted into your torso, with your belly drawn in and your back rounded.

Step 4 On your inhale, reextend your right leg back into a Downward Dog split behind you.

Step 5 On your next exhale, bend your right knee and draw it toward the outside of your right arm, above the floor. Keep your knee and leg lifted, with your belly drawn in.

Step 6 On your next inhale, reextend your leg back to the Downward Dog split behind you.

Step 7 On your next exhale, bend your right knee and draw it across your midline to the outside of your left wrist. You will be twisting. Keep your knee and leg lifted, and your belly drawn in.

Step 8 On your next inhale, reextend your leg back into a Downward Dog split, and then to the floor, to meet your left foot. Rest. Repeat on the left side.

THINGS TO THINKABOUT
- Feel free to lower your left knee to the floor and work from the Table pose. Over time, start to build up and see if you can do just the beginning in the Downward Dog.

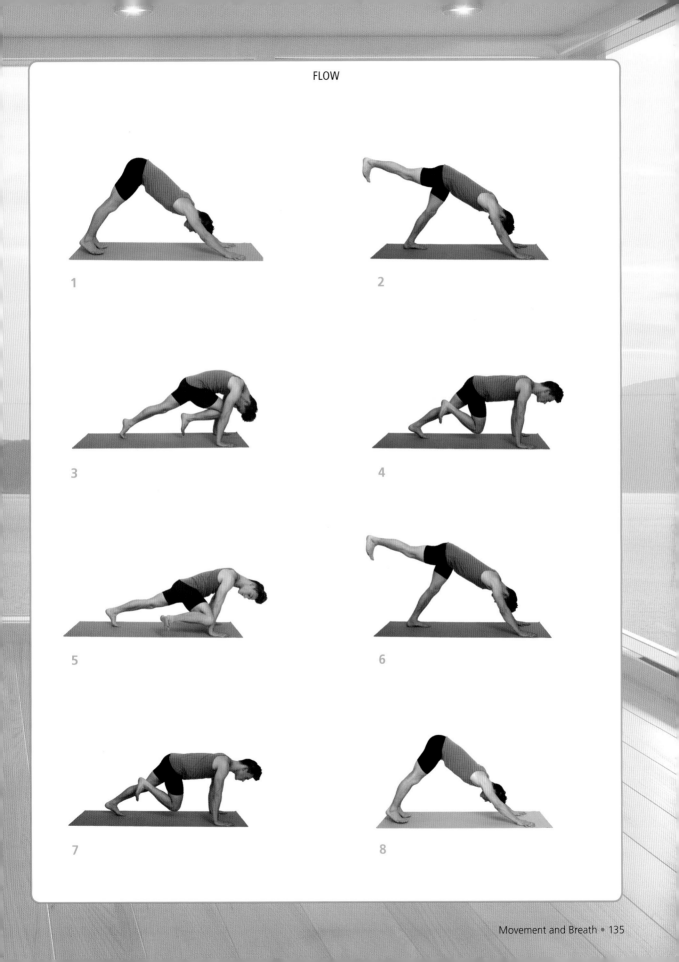

1

2

3

4

5

6

7

8

Warrior II Flow

Step 1 Start in the Warrior II pose (page 32), and turn your palms up. On your next inhale, straighten your front leg, lift your arms up over your head, bring your palms together, and look up.

Step 2 On your exhale, bend your front knee over your ankle, stretch your arms out to the sides, and end with them at shoulder height, palms down. Look out over your left hand.

Step 3 Inhale, exhale, and then release your front forearm to your thigh. Move into the Extended Side Angle pose. Extend your top arm, palm up overhead, alongside your ear.

Step 4 Inhale and flow back through the Warrior II pose. On your exhale, come into the Reverse Warrior pose—keeping your front knee bent. Release your back palm to your back thigh and lift the opposite arm. Gaze at your lifted hand.

Step 5 Inhale and return to the Warrior II pose.

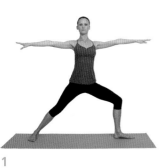

1

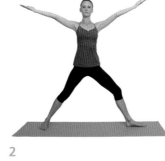

2

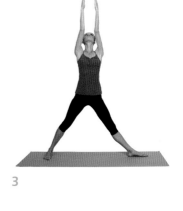

3

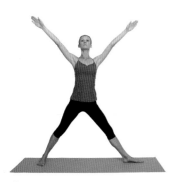

4

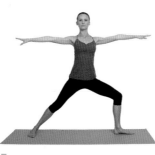

5

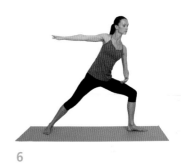

6

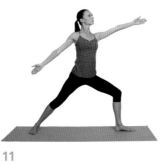

7

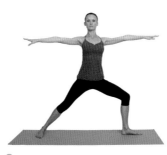

8

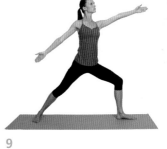

9

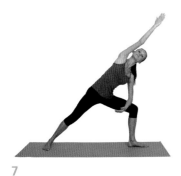

10

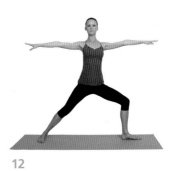

11

12

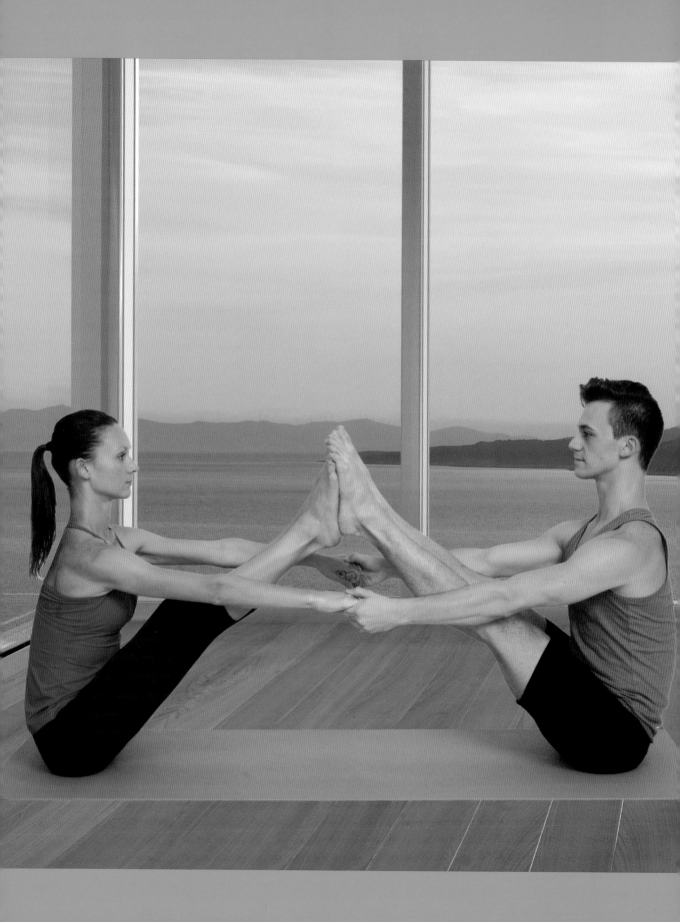

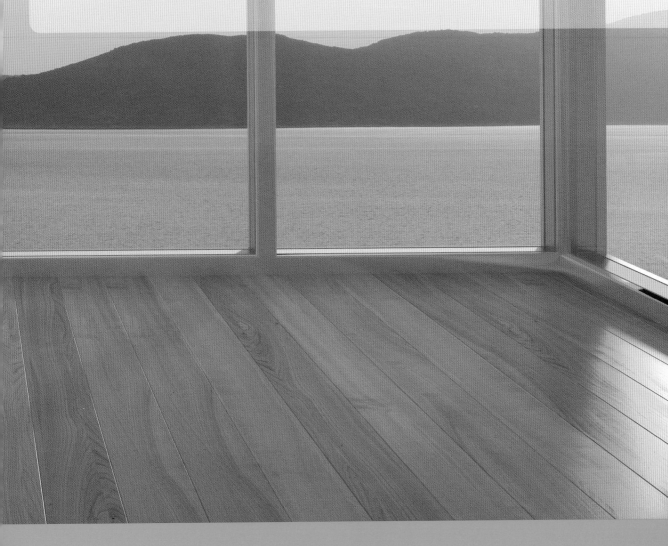

Partner Yoga

Partner yoga is a fun way to practice together. Incorporate each other's bodies to create stability and structure in your yoga poses. You may find it easier to move deeper, hold a pose longer, and balance when working with a partner than when practicing by yourself. Stay focused on each other, your movements, and your breath.

Double Seated
Sukasana

This very simple partner yoga pose is the perfect way to start and end a practice.

Step 1 Sit comfortably back to back. Decide if you need a blanket to sit on, and if so, both of you should sit on the same height prop.

Step 2 Notice if your backs feel balanced right to left, and assess if you are leaning more forward or back. Communicate as you both make the adjustments to feel as balanced as possible.

Step 3 Notice your body touching your partner's body. Where is there contact? Do you feel supported?

Step 4 Bring awareness to the lower part of your body first. Relax your feet, legs, and hips into the floor. Keep your spine lifted, but allow for the skin on your back to relax down. Feel the top of your shoulders drop and your arms and hands let go.

Step 5 Find the length in your neck, and notice if your head is balanced over your tailbone.

Step 6 Release your jaw, teeth, and tongue. Soften your eyes and feel your eyelids relax over your eyeballs.

Step 7 Notice your breath. Consciously watch your inhale and exhale, allowing it to be just what it is at this moment. Be with your breath.

THINGS TO THINK ABOUT
- Notice if you can feel your partner breathing against your back. Can you feel any type of sensation, as their back expands and contracts with each breath?
- Notice anything that is similar or different about the two breaths. Watch yourself and your partner breathing.
- Go back to noticing the support of your partner's body and enjoy this moment of ease.

Double Upward-Facing Boat Pose
Paripurna Navasana

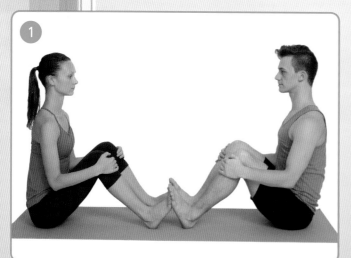

Step 1 Sit facing your partner. Keep your knees bent, and bring the soles of your feet together.

Step 2 Take hold of each other's hands. Keep your lower back lifted, with the top of your shoulders soft and down.

Step 3 Press into the sole of your partner's foot, and slowly lift and straighten that leg. Do the same on the other.

Step 4 Keep your toes pointed up, with your legs and arms extended.

Step 5 Lift your lower back, open your chest, and breathe consciously together.

Step 6 After a few breaths, lower one leg to the floor at a time, release your hands, and sit relaxed on the floor.

3

Double King Dancer
Natarajasana

Step 1 Stand 3-4 feet apart, facing each other. Join your corresponding palms—your right palm and your partner's left, or vice versa. Lift your corresponding arms and press your palms into each other for support.

Step 2 Lift and bend the other corresponding leg and hold the outside of your ankle.

Step 3 Press into your partner's palm, and kick your foot into your hand, lifting your leg behind you.

Step 4 The key to this pose is to move forward and back at the same time. Use your partner's help to stabilize you.

Step 5 You can lift your back leg higher by arching further forward, which will also help to better keep your balance.

Step 6 Enjoy the sense of ease and freedom in this pose that you can find only with a partner.

Step 7 Release this pose consciously, together, and at the same time.

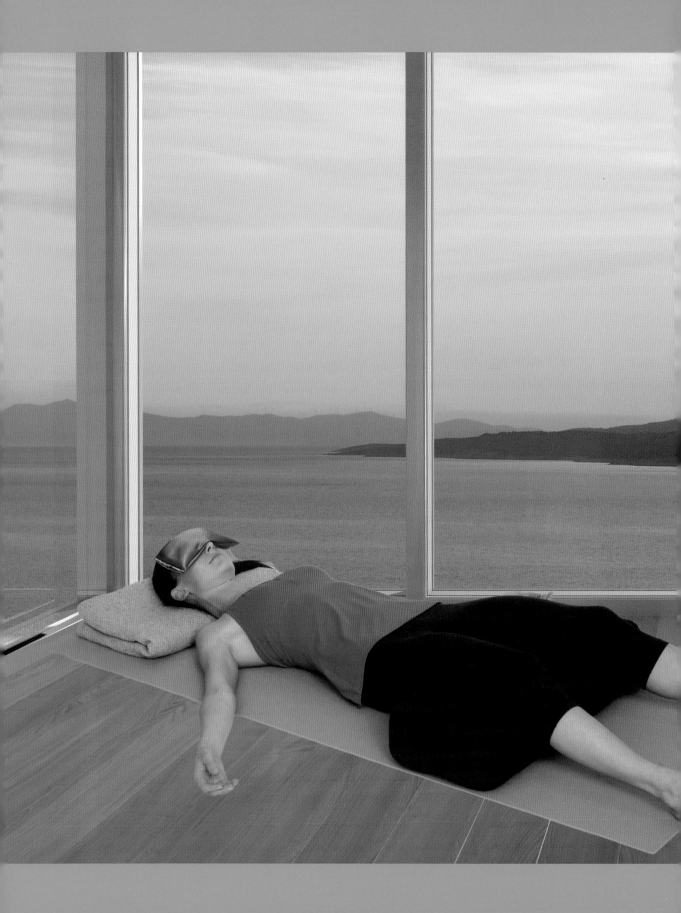

Relaxation, Breath, and Meditation

When we talk about relaxation in yoga class, it is different than lounging on the couch watching TV. Most Westerners believe that yoga is the practice of the asanas (postures), but the asanas were originally taught as a preparation so that students could sit comfortably for meditation. How many of us can simply plop down with our legs crossed, sit up straight, close our eyes, and hold still for 30 minutes? Not many. So the poses and relaxation techniques were developed to bring balance to the body, and the breathing practices enabled students to finally sit for meditation. So the next time you want to slip out before this part of class, or think that you don't have time to do this in your living room, realize that you could be missing out on some of the most profound benefits of a complete practice.

Breathing Practices
Pranayama

Breathing practices were developed to enhance the physical awareness of how we breathe. You may question at first why you need to be taught how to breathe. We breathe in and out—what's the big deal? But in daily life when we are anxious, hurried, or stressed, our breathing follows. We get in the habit of shallow, constricted breathing, likely not even realizing until we walk into class and are instructed to consciously take a full, deep breath. As the nervous system rebalances and our minds learn how to focus, we have the ability to realize the full range of our breathing potential. With full deep breaths, the diaphragm muscle moves up and down, pulling, tugging, and pushing, not only on the lungs but also all the other internal organs around the lungs. This push and pull is like a big massage to the organs, keeping the blood flowing and the organs healthy. Also, full deep breaths use the bottom part of the lungs, which we rarely inhale or exhale from consciously. Breathing also moves the lymph around your body. Lymph is part of your immune system, which fights infection and detoxifies the body.

The great thing about breathing practice is, with practice, you can do it anywhere. Stuck in traffic, overwhelmed at work, arguing with the kids? You will find that being able to control your breathing will help you manage the situation in a healthier way.

Full Complete Breaths

Sitting or lying down comfortably, support your body so the sensations of your body begin to quiet down. Take the time to do this. Remember to breathe in and out through your nose, unless you can't breathe easily. Begin by closing your eyes and just watch how you are breathing at this moment.

Ask yourself some questions: What is the quality of my breathing right now? Is it slow or fast? Deep or shallow? But don't try to change it yet. Just watch. After about a minute or so, begin to breathe in deeper.

Can you break up your breathing into three parts? Take in a third of your breath capacity, then the second third, and then all of it. You should be at the top of the breath. And then begin to exhale, doing so with a full, complete exhalation.

As you watch yourself do this, is it easy or hard, interesting or boring? Whatever it is, can you just continue to be present, watching yourself and your breath?

If you find yourself distracted, the moment you realize it, just bring yourself back to the full, complete breath. This distraction is going to happen many times, but that doesn't matter. Just keep bringing yourself back to the flow of the breath. See if you can start with full, complete breathing for a minute or two. Then return to your natural breathing and notice how you feel.

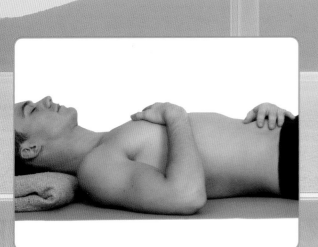
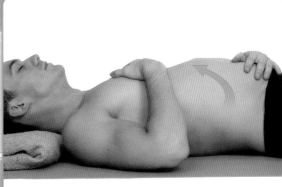

Alternate Nostril Breathing
Nadhi Sudi

Sit up in a comfortable position—lean against the wall if needed. Begin by bringing your awareness to your natural breathing. Then curl the index and middle finger of your right hand into your palm. This is known as Vishnu Mudra.

Use your thumb to close your right nostril, and your ring finger and pinky finger to close your left nostril. With your left nostril closed, inhale through your right nostril, then close the right and open the left. Exhale out the left, inhale, close the left, open the right, and exhale.

Continue with a gentle, calm breath. Now lengthen the exhalation 2-3 seconds longer than the inhalation. Eventually lengthen the exhalation to twice as long as the inhalation.

At the beginning, try this practice for 10 cycles, then return to your natural breathing. Remember not to pinch the nose; a gentle press of your nostril is all that is needed.

If you become anxious practicing this or any other breathing practice, bring yourself back to your natural breathing pattern.

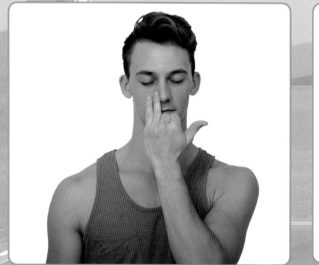 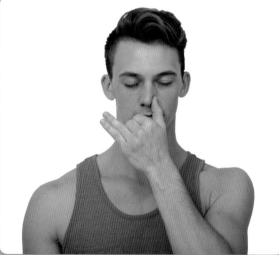

Meditation

The word "meditation" conjures up images of monks sitting on the floor. Classic meditation is practiced sitting in a cross-legged position on the floor with your eyes closed, being still. As discussed before, sitting is challenging for Westerners, and having full attention on the present moment is an even bigger challenge. So, the practice of meditation can be adapted to be done with movement. Maybe you are a swimmer or runner. Can you stay conscious as you do this repetitive movement? Can you watch your arms and legs move over and over again? Can you count the movements, continue to watch the movements, and stay present? If a thought comes up unrelated to this repetitive movement, can you put it off to the side for later? The process of watching your body, breathing, and thoughts is the practice of meditation. We don't accomplish meditation, we practice it. It is always a practice—it may be easier some days and harder on others, but basically the idea is to develop this focus over time. At first you may find that your yoga practice, moving from pose to pose, can be the tool you use for your meditation practice. Any time you draw your attention to the present moment, your breathing, and your body, you are meditating. Keep trying this practice during different daily activities—eating, washing the dishes, folding the laundry, and walking down the street. The more you do it, the easier it gets.

Step 1 Sit on a folded blanket on the floor.

Step 2 Bend your knees, crossing your legs at the shins.

Step 3 Your knees should rest comfortably below your hips. Sit up higher on folded blankets if this alignment does not come naturally. If it is challenging to sit up, place the blanket up against a wall and sit back with the wall to support you.

Step 4 Feel your buttock bones ground into the mat or blankets as you lift through your spine and the crown of your head.

Step 5 Move your upper arms back to open your chest.

Step 6 Simply bring your awareness to your breathing, watch it move in and out of your nose without effort. Allow your thoughts to move through your mind.

Step 7 If you find yourself getting lost, simply bring yourself back to the sensations in your body, and the movement of your breath flowing in and out of your body. Nothing more, nothing less.

Supine Bound Angle Pose
Supta Baddhakonasana

This pose can be practiced by anyone, but it is especially helpful for women who are pregnant, menstruating, or menopausal. A deep state of relaxation takes place here. Propping is imperative to stay in the pose comfortably. Cover yourself with a blanket to stay warm.

Step 1 Prepare your setup by propping a bolster up on a block. Have three or four blankets handy.

Step 2 Sit just in front of the bolster with the soles of your feet together.

Step 3 Gently lie back on the bolster.

Step 4 If your knees don't reach the floor, or if there is too deep a stretch in the groin, prop your knees up with blankets or blocks.

Step 5 Let your arms rest at your sides, palms up.

Corpse Pose
Savasana

This is the icing on the cake. Every yoga practice should end with the Corpse pose, even if it is only a couple of minutes long. Prop your body so it is completely comfortable, balanced, and even. Only then can the nervous system become quiet. This pose allows you the time to incorporate the benefits of your practice: mind, body, and spirit.

Step 1 Lie on your back, with your legs extended. If your lower back is sensitive, place a bolster or folded blanket under your thighs.

Step 2 Allow your legs and feet to fall open.

Step 3 Let your arms rest alongside your body, allowing some space between your torso and arms, palms facing up.

Step 4 Gently turn your head from side to side, finding the natural point for your skull to rest.

Step 5 As you let your breath flow naturally, sequentially relax all of the muscles of your body, from your toes to your face.

Step 6 Come out of the pose by drawing your knees to your chest, pause, then roll to one side, pause, and come back to a seated position, head last.

Workouts

During yoga classes, the teacher instructs students through a series of poses. These poses are "linked" together, either by a specific order: from simpler poses to more advanced poses, a focus on one type of pose (such as back bends), or with the even flow of your breath. Once you become more familiar with the poses, your can choose a series of poses that "flow" well together, feel good in your body, and either challenge or relax you, depending on your mood that day. Following are a couple of pose flows that you may experiment with. They start simple and increase in difficulty. Remember to listen to your body, follow your energy, begin to coordinate and lengthen your breath with your movements, and know that you will feel more balanced and lighter at the end of the practice. Feel free to modify or eliminate any pose at any time. It is always important to start with sitting, grounding and settling yourself, connecting with your breath before you begin warm-ups. Coming full circle, end with a long, satisfying deep relaxation (Corpse pose, page 153). Give yourself at least 5-15 minutes. The Corpse pose is the time to integrate the benefits of the poses you just completed.

Simple Pose Flow 15-30 minutes

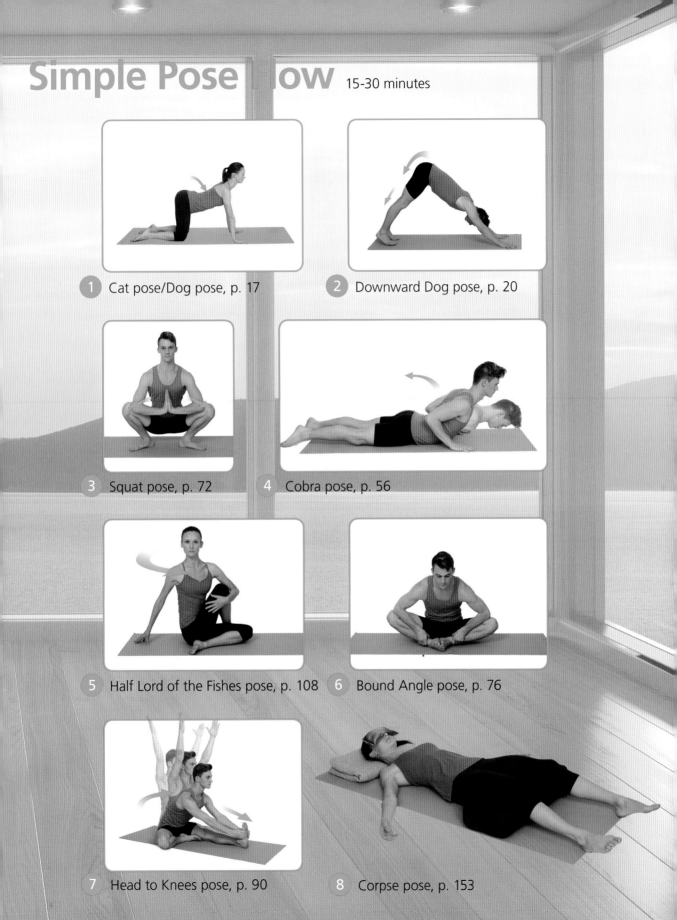

1 Cat pose/Dog pose, p. 17

2 Downward Dog pose, p. 20

3 Squat pose, p. 72

4 Cobra pose, p. 56

5 Half Lord of the Fishes pose, p. 108

6 Bound Angle pose, p. 76

7 Head to Knees pose, p. 90

8 Corpse pose, p. 153

Gentle Flow 45-60 minutes

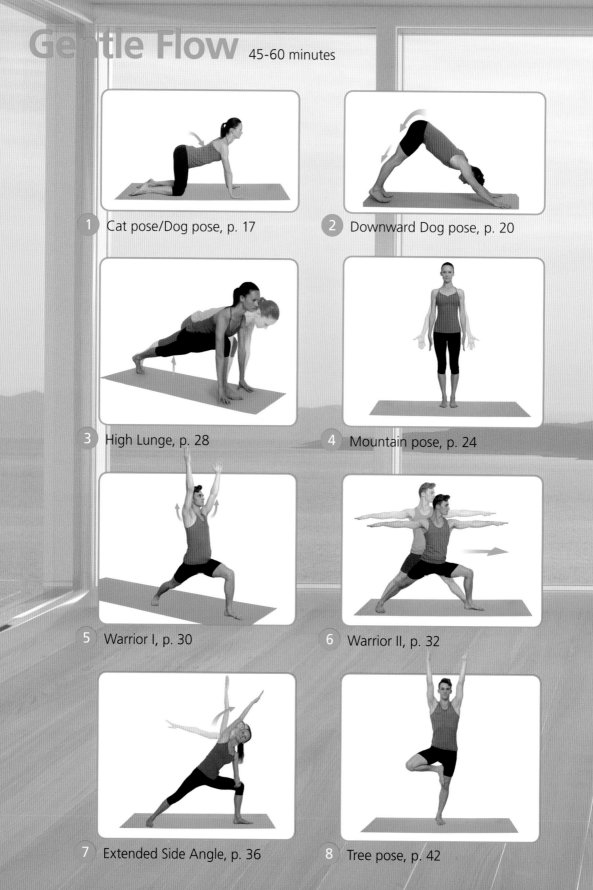

1. Cat pose/Dog pose, p. 17

2. Downward Dog pose, p. 20

3. High Lunge, p. 28

4. Mountain pose, p. 24

5. Warrior I, p. 30

6. Warrior II, p. 32

7. Extended Side Angle, p. 36

8. Tree pose, p. 42

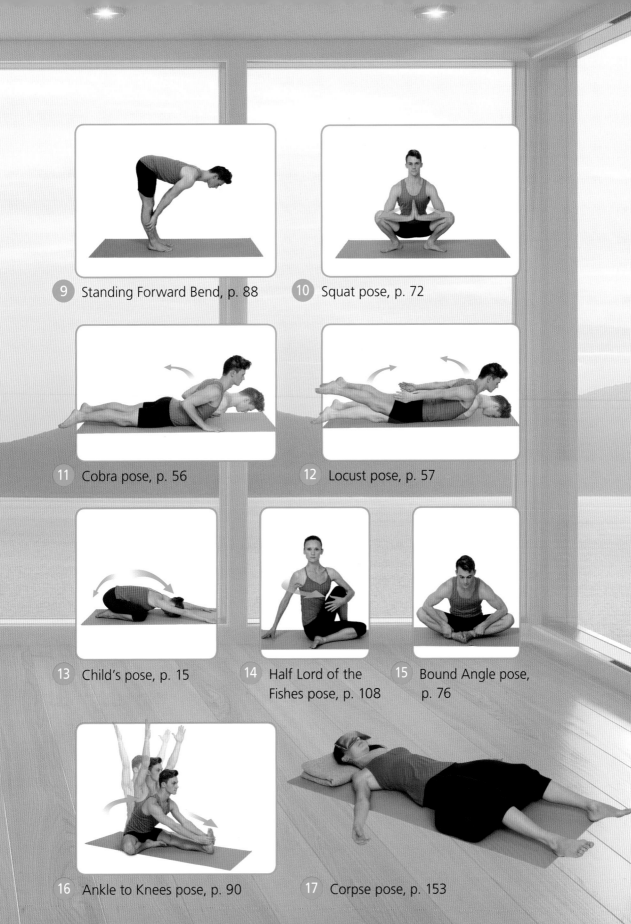

9 Standing Forward Bend, p. 88

10 Squat pose, p. 72

11 Cobra pose, p. 56

12 Locust pose, p. 57

13 Child's pose, p. 15

14 Half Lord of the
Fishes pose, p. 108

15 Bound Angle pose,
p. 76

16 Ankle to Knees pose, p. 90

17 Corpse pose, p. 153

Energized Flow 45-60 minutes

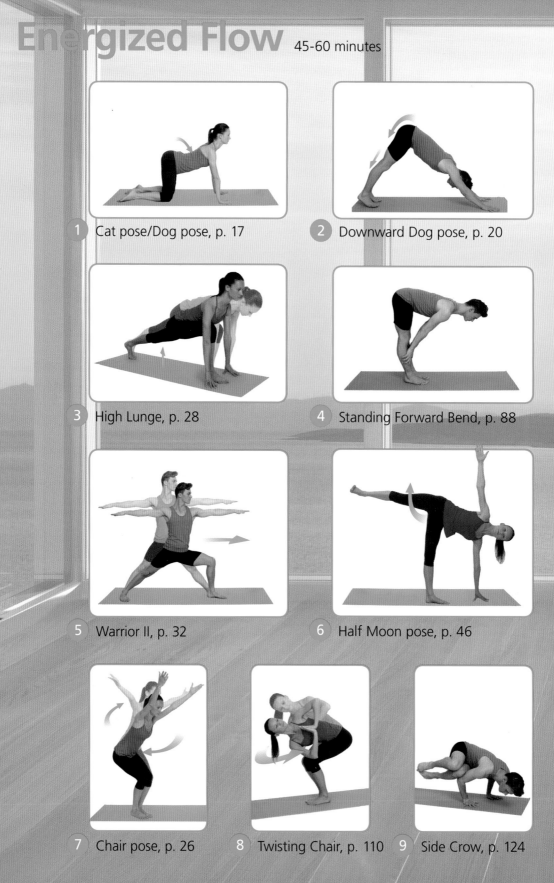

1 Cat pose/Dog pose, p. 17

2 Downward Dog pose, p. 20

3 High Lunge, p. 28

4 Standing Forward Bend, p. 88

5 Warrior II, p. 32

6 Half Moon pose, p. 46

7 Chair pose, p. 26

8 Twisting Chair, p. 110

9 Side Crow, p. 124

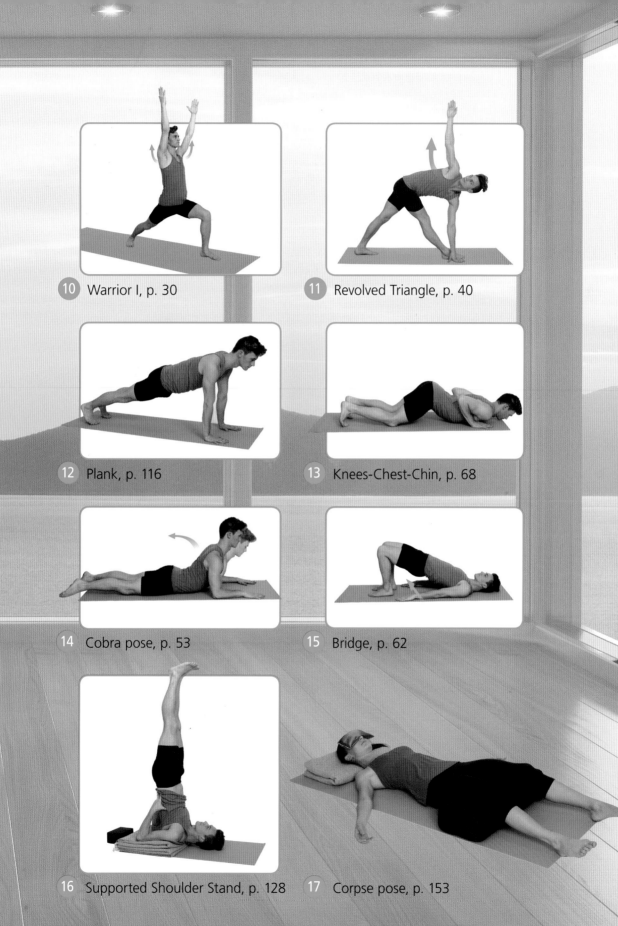

10 Warrior I, p. 30

11 Revolved Triangle, p. 40

12 Plank, p. 116

13 Knees-Chest-Chin, p. 68

14 Cobra pose, p. 53

15 Bridge, p. 62

16 Supported Shoulder Stand, p. 128

17 Corpse pose, p. 153

Acknowledgments

Photography

Photography by Jonathan Conklin

www.jonathanconklin.net

Illustrations

All illustrations by Hector Aiza/3D Labz Animation India, except pages 6 and 7 and the insets on pages 10, 11, 15, 16, 18, 30, 37, 39, 42, 43, 45, 46, 76, 77, 84, 85, 86, 87, 94, 99, 100, 109, 110, 111, 112, 114, 115, 116, 117, 121, 122, 123, 124, 125, 128, 129, 130, 131, 132, 133, 138, 148: by Shutterstock/Linda Bucklin.